Ditch The Diet
Dare To Define

A book that translates customary diet culture to a
contemporary yet rooted intuitive eating.

a NutritionOnUrPlate Initiative

© Compiled by Preetha Kkiran

NOTION PRESS

NOTION PRESS

India. Singapore. Malaysia.

युक्ताहारविहारस्य युक्तचेष्टस्य कर्मसु ।
युक्तस्वप्नावबोधस्य योगो भवति दुःखहा ।।

yuktāhāra-vihārasya yukta-cheṣṭasya karmasu

yukta-svapnāvabodhasya yogo bhavati duḥkha-hā

"The one, whose diet and movements are balanced,
whose actions are proper, whose hours of sleeping
and waking up are regular,
and who follows the path of meditation,
is the destroyer of pain or unhappiness."

- *Lord Krishna, Gita*
Chapter 6 Shloka 17

*This book is a tribute to my father **Mr. P. S. V. Subramanian** who at 82 years of age is a paragon of a healthy lifestyle relying on strongly rooted thoughts of Ayurveda and Intuitive Eating. He has been my role model and inspiration in serving and contributing through my experience and expertise in nutrition to society at large.*

*This book is only possible due to the support of my family, especially my daughter, a psychologist in the making, **Ms. Keyosha Kiran Anchan**, whose valuable inputs are much cherished.*

*My husband, a master mariner, **Capt. Kiran Anchan** has, in his own unique way rendered all his support to everything that I wanted to indulge in, to stand by me with his assurance when I needed to be fearless and plunge in to reach the little milestones of my life.*

*My son, a teenager, a sports enthusiast and a budding footballer, **Mstr. Yuvansh Kiran Anchan** has been that spark of careless cheer and necessary distraction from the daily routines.*

*My brother, a corporate manager, **Mr Shankar Raman** whom I completely admire for his relentless support and love. and his better half, a pharmacist by profession, **Ms Lakshmi Shankar Raman** whose kindness make our family's life better along with our international financial advisor **Mr Aaditya Shankar Raman**, my nephew and my niece **Ms. Aarya Shankar Raman**, a promising future business consultant, all of whom have been very patient and understanding considering the time I have spent compiling this book,*

*My Mother-in-law **Ms. Anju Kumar**, a formidable and dynamic personality herself, who taught me to be fearless and focused.*

*Last but not least, our dear playful pawed pet **King Kaylo**, a Rottie whose unconditional love helped me easily sail through this journey.*

"There are no shortcuts to any place worth going, it is you my dear family who held hands and walked along this path for my dreams."

Contents

CONTENTS

Foreword

Preetha Kkiran is a renowned nutritionist based in Mumbai, with expertise over 23 years in the field of nutrition. She manages her platform, *NutritionOnUrPlate*, both online and offline, professionally helping the development of a healthy lifestyle. She is a passionate and knowledgeable professional engaged in various aspects of the wellness industry.

Preetha's specialization includes genomics, obesity management, beauty, wellness, skin and haircare services. Her research efforts on nutrition interventions in healthcare have helped her develop a unique approach to coaching individuals thereby positively impacting their lives. Her commitment is unparalleled in traditional circles when it comes to providing personalized nutritional attention to each of her clients.

Preetha holds a Master's degree in food science and nutrition, and is currently a PhD student with UGC and Ayurveda Master certificate course pupil. She also holds a diploma in Cosmetology Laser Skin Hair Aesthetics from Artistry pro academy (Mumbai) and certifications from IDA (Indian Dietetics Association), IAPEN (India), and DHA (UAE). She is a life member of IDA and holds certifications in Public Health Nutrition (UK), Role of Diabetes Educator (UK), Certified Diabetic Educator (India), and Certified Nutrigenomics expert (India).

Preetha's career path includes working in multinational companies like Cadbury India, Britannia and co, during her graduation and post-graduation studies. She has also worked with VLCC Healthcare, VLCC International LLC, Maricos Group, Al Futtaim, KYP Holistic LLC, Godrej Group and Aeroflex Industries, among others, that has contributed greatly to her professional techniques.

Overall, Preetha is a trailblazer, dedicated to continuous learning and upgrading her skills.

Additionally, she is a corporate wellness consultant, & conducts numerous webinars and workshops in her daily work routine. Preetha Kkiran is capable of offering wellness services to all employees in your esteemed organization. These encompass the following parameters:

- BCA – Segmental Analysis (Inbody)

- Anthropometry – Body Measurements, Height and Waist Circumference, BMI

- Fitness Evaluation – Posture & Flexibility

- Analysis of Skin and Hair – One-on-one Analysis

- Physical Condition – Questionnaire & Discussion

- Medical Condition – Profiles of Blood & Urine tests

- Lifestyle – Availability of Time and Work Schedule

- DNA (Genome) Screening – Personalised (precision) Diet & Exercise Regimen

- Evaluating Stress Management – Personal Questionnaire

Happiness is homemade.

Neha Sawant

Author of "SALES VUE" & Sales Expert

Date: September 5th, 2023

Preface

Time to ***Ditch the Diet; Dare to Define***

NutritionOnUrPlate stands for developing consumer attitude that rejects fast fixes and embraces a more holistic approach to health, viewing food as loving, nourishing, and therapeutic. You can leverage food and drink to avoid health issues by modifying your eating habits in the same manner that you would use any latest technology or tool. This is based on a concept developed by my team and me, that was initially investigated in our 2015 endeavour, Know your Persona Holistic Center LLC, UAE.

We need to enhance health where it begins, within us, where we live, work, eat, sleep, study, and play. The anti-diet attitude, proactive approach to food intake, and holistic approach to well-being springs from life lessons learnt from my journey as a nutritionist to an entrepreneur.

We are connected by studies into both mental and physical wellness as well as by choosing to follow the most reliable, certified, experienced healthcare professionals when choosing the design of your program. Contrary to any conventional diet concept, *NutritionOnUrPlate* centres on food and drink selections from a variety of sources, through medical tests, body composition, genetic tests, family history, lifestyle, allergies, intolerances, likes, dislikes as well as an individual's willingness towards the program.

Personally, I eat more instinctively and pay attention to what my body is telling me. I would indulge myself with Italian cuisines without going overboard while I was expecting; I never followed a diet per-se, and have always been a little sceptic when I hear about a trending diet or trend. As a nutritionist, I understand true gluten sensitivity, but I also find that the majority of gluten-free food items are merely fashion statements. I believe that if you don't have any allergies or intolerances, you shouldn't need to avoid gluten. My formative years have served me well to gather the bulk of knowledge pertaining to food and drink being passed down indigenously. My Master's degree in Food Science and Nutrition at SNDT University served to reinforce things that I had learned growing up. This was further established during my years (23 or so, at the time of writing this) of experience in the health sector, with routine online research, reading a number of relevant books on nutrition, and by engaging with several professional mentors who encouraged me while I was in different roles – a student, an employee, an entrepreneur, founder and a wellness speaker.

I must state this clearly, and perhaps boldly too, through this book – Lots of fads emerging in the market only serve to lure individuals into false assurances and fleecing unsuspecting folks just to make a quick buck out of them. I believe that one must consume things that are in season and healthy. While, I appreciate the study on probiotics, I disagree that blindly adding kimchi or sauerkraut to our regular meals or drinking kombucha is a good idea, beyond serving to keep up with the popular craze.

When choosing what to eat, I believe it is crucial to consider our own food systems and cultural cuisines. I would be content to consume curd rice and fermented pickles, but only if they complement the rest of my diet and provide me with the necessary probiotics. In light of this, I would conclude by stating that no one book can convey all knowledge and that this book is neither flawless nor comprehensive. If this book inspires every generation of young nutritionists to re-evaluate their approach to life as humans, health, and nutrition from a fresh perspective, that would be my genuine reward.

Preetha Kkiran

Date: August 24th, 2023

Acknowledgments

No acknowledgement would not be befitting, if I missed out on a thank you note to **Ms. Vandana Luthra**, VLCC group of companies, who through her thought process built an empire and simultaneously redefined the lives of many women including yours truly. Thank you for changing the trajectory of my career for the better. I can never truly express how grateful I am.

I would want to thank *Perippa* **Mr. P.K. Venkatraman** for being a wonderful influence and a great mentor right throughout my childhood. It is your appreciation that I longed for, the most, in every small little accomplishment as a little girl. To love something that you do wholeheartedly is what I learnt from you. Your interest in minute details; to notice and appreciate the things that we often take for granted are huge life lessons for me.

Mr. Yusuf Kagzi MD, Aeroflex Industries LTD, who readily supports me in all my initiatives and renders his expertise for the enhancement of the same.

My deepest gratitude to the entire team of *NutritionOnUrPlate*, previously KYP Holistic Center LLC, **Ms. Deepali Vinod, Dr. Suheba Tabassum** Physiotherapy, **Ms. Shella, Ms. Rizza, Ms. Marinell, Ms. Reetu, Ms. Rodalyne, Ms. Asra Sheikh, Ms. Anita Jijimon**. Thank you for always inspiring me to put my best foot forward.

A hearty thanks to my dearest friend & fellow nutritionist **Ms. Swati Chandrashekar** founder, Celebrity Nutritionist, and a Ph.D. Scholar, Pune.

I would like to thank my mentor and guide, a dear friend, entrepreneur, author & influencer, Founder of SawantBazaar.com, Founder – Nexplore, **Ms. Neha Sawant**, of whom I will remain ever so grateful, for her persuasion, constant encouragement, and motivation to compile this book, and whose invaluable contributions and inputs have made this book an interesting read.

Heartfelt thanks to **Mr. Yogesh M.A.** – Digital Leadership Trainer for his immense trust in my abilities and **Ms. Khushboo Chotaliya,** author, Founder of Sanskari Decor, for her patient reading, timely feedback, and valuable inputs and constant support.

The OHC dept of Aeroflex **Ms. Trupti** – HR staff welfare, **Ms. Asmita** – Head nurse OHC, **Mr. Hari** – Safety office, **Mr. Jitesh Bhoir** – Supervisor, and **Mr. Chetan Bhoir** – HR head, have helped make this book possible through their readiness, I am a wiser person because of those insightful sessions.

I extend my gratitude to **Dr. Mala Pandurang**, Principal of BMN College, your dedication continues to amaze and inspire me to put in that little more effort, I hope to make you proud.

Ms. Anuradha Shekar Retd. Professor, Nutrition Dept of BMN College thank you for seeing potential in me and helping me harness it. Your recommendations have always given me the zeal and confidence to excel; and **Dr. Shobha Udipi** Retd. HOD, Food Science and Nutrition SNDT (Juhu) for stimulating my interest in the subject of nutrition and constantly keeping me captivated to this wonderful area or work, kindling my passion and motivating me to carve a successful career out of it.

Dr. Jagdip Shah – Gynaecologist, obstetrician, who introduced me to Aesthetics, thank you for showing me what true work ethics and work-life balance are.

Dr. Manish Motwani – Gastroenterologist, bariatric surgeon, I can't think of a better way to describe your gentle but firm support through my career changes. All the counselling outside of our sessions has made me a better person. Indeed, fortunate to have met you.

Dr. Kirti Samudra – Diabetologist **Dr Mohan's** Diabetic Clinic, I am glad to have you in my corner.

Dr. Prattusha – Ph.D. Scholar Onco Psychology, **Dr. Nirali** – Physiotherapist, **Dr. Ravindra Jain** – General Health & **Dr. Sujata Ghawi, Dr. Aparna Pandya** Chaitali Polyclinic, for contributing relevant and interesting aspects and setting examples through your practice that helped shape the chapters in this book.

Ms. Meera Menezes – Ex HR Sun Microsystems, Ex Coordinator Orchids, The International School, my dearest friend; your constant reassurance has helped me navigate through tough times.

And a little shoutout to her hubby **Mr. Alvin Menezes – CTO, Calculus Systems Pvt. Ltd.** who also happens to be my childhood friend because of whom I strive to excel in every tiny step I take. You raise my bar buddy.

Ms. Niddhi Khanna – Ex Head Trainer Soft Skills Centum Learning and Development, your direction and insightful comments have made me a better professional.

Ms. Aman Kawar – Ex VP of VLCC INDIA, who has favoured me beyond my wildest imagination. Thank you for being a caring, loving and dedicated mentor in every way.

Ms. Sushma Patil – MD ArtistryPro Beauty Training Institute without your help, I wouldn't be exposed to so many opportunities.

Sincere gratitude to all my mentors, friends, fraternity, clients, colleagues, associates, and well-wishers who have been a huge support throughout the years and have inspired me to do better work.

Enjoy the experience.

Introduction

"Writing this book has been even more satisfying than I had anticipated."

The idea of putting this book together sprouted as a challenge to the frequent apprehensions and reservations that I had in my practice as a nutritionist for over 23 years. Following the trends and banal methods of addressing health and obesity management through different dietary approaches, reluctantly following guidelines that were designed in a not-so-similar environment acted as a catalyst towards this initiative. I needed to share my learnings from a practical perspective to better one's life through the tools I had amassed throughout. I had put these into use since long past to help transform the lives of individuals in need of guidance.

As individuals or professionals, we are always looking for new and better ways to maintain our health, whether it be through technology or diet. Over the years, the diet industry has experienced massive growth. Like any other aspect of our culture, our diet constantly changes and evolves. However, with the rise of social media, dieting and exercising have become a culture in itself.

So why do diet culture norms seem to change every so often? Are the claims really sustainable? Do we thoroughly research the diet or product that we are buying and ensure that it is intended to efficiently and safely deliver claimed results?

Consumers have a right to make informed choices in today's fast-paced world. Today, we are a lot less active than we were in the past. We walk a lot less and do less physical work. We snack more and consume a growing number of calories from sugary drinks, crisps and chocolate. We also eat a lot more processed foods, which are notoriously high in sugar and salt.

Whilst on my initial research I stumbled upon the facts that were alarming like

- Consumption of semi-skimmed milk overtook whole milk in 1993.

- Bananas replaced apples as the most popular fruit in 1996.

- We drink 12 times as much bottled water now as we did in the 1980s.

- According to the survey, we purchase 75% less white bread today than we did in 1974, and 85% more brown and wholemeal bread.

- Consumption of eggs peaked in the 1960s and has been declining ever since.

- We buy fewer carrots, turnips, parsnips, cabbages and sprouts than the previous generation.

We are all into **Sustainable eating** that does not question the person. Instead, it questions the food source, consumption pattern, and eating attitudes. However, that has not helped us achieve the ultimate goal of a healthy life and that is where **Intuitive Eating** comes into play. It does not question the food source, it rather questions the person eating the meal, the mindset behind each meal.

Through this book, I have made it my mission to blend our age-old practices of *Ayurveda* with **Intuitive Eating** by trusting one's body to make food choices that feel good without judging yourself or the influence of diet.

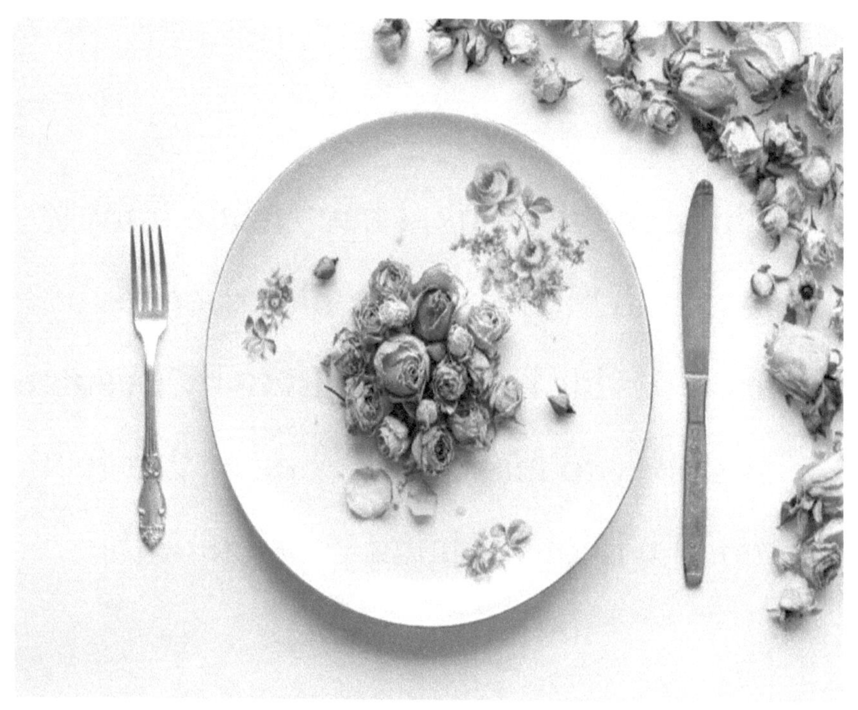

Intuitive Eating Initiative

Value the food you eat

पूजितं ह्यशनं नित्यं बलमूर्जं च यच्छति ।

अपूजितं तु तद् भुक्तमुभयं नाशयेदिदम् ॥

pūjitaṃ hyaśanaṃ nityaṃ balamūrjaṃ ca yacchati

apūjitaṃ tu tad bhuktamubhayaṃ nāśayedidam

"Food partaken of with reverence results in strength and longevity,
and the destruction of both, when partaken of irreverently."

\-   *Manusmriti 2/55*

1. Diet

Foxcroft asserts that the word "diet" is derived from the Greek word *diaita*, which connotes a sense of an all-encompassing healthy lifestyle, involving both mental and physical health, as opposed to a specific weight-loss program.

Ancient Indians consumed a diet comprising mostly of wheat, barley, vegetables, fruits (Indian dates, mangoes, and berries), meats (cow, sheep and goats), and dairy products. Archaeologists have found fishing nets and hooks in the ruins of early Indian civilizations, showing that they also liked to catch and eat fish; they grew rice, peas, sesame, and melons. And they domesticated cows, pigs, buffalo, and sheep. They cooked using clay ovens, cauldrons, and open fires. And they knew how to dry and pickle food to preserve it.

If you visited someone in early India, you would most likely be served rice, veggies, meat, and wheat bread. There would be a marked difference depending on the region though. In the north, they tended to eat food that was more bland (not spicy), with a lot of dairy products (yogurt and butter), and lentils. In the south, you would find the food a tad spicier, and served with rice and perhaps coconut. Those who lived near the oceans, rivers, or lakes would serve fish and seafood.

Later on, religion began to influence what food was eaten. The Hindus came to see the cow as a sacred animal, and would not eat it. Muslims were forbidden to eat pork as well. And though India had learned about chickens from Thailand and sheep from the Middle East, a section of the populace chose to be vegetarians, rather than associate with the guilt of slaughtering animals.

Food was seen as important to a person's holiness. There were many rules and rituals regarding food. For example, people were forbidden from eating carnivorous (animals that eat meat) animals, and from eating garlic. It was believed that a person's mind was affected by his nutrition, so this was taken very seriously.

Traditional Indian foods have been prepared for many years and preparation varies across the country. Time-honoured wisdom about processing of food, its preservation techniques, and their therapeutic effects have been established for many generations in India. Food systems can deliver numerous biological functions through dietary components in the human body. Indian traditional foods are also recognized as functional foods because of the presence of functional components such as body-healing chemicals, antioxidants, dietary fibres, and probiotics. These functional molecules help in weight management, and blood sugar level balance and support immunity of the body. The functional properties of foods are further enhanced by processing techniques such as sprouting, malting, and fermentation.

According to Aryan belief, food was considered as a source of strength and a gift from God. Aryans believed that food was not simply meant for body nourishment, but was the basic part of a cosmic moral cycle.

Ayurveda is a traditional system of medicines native to India. In *Ayurveda*, regulation of diet is crucial, since it examines the whole human body as the product of food. Food is responsible for different aspects of an individual including physical, temperamental, and mental states. Based on the dominant constituent of the body, doshas are classified into *kapha*, *pitta*, and *vatta*. *Ayurveda*, not only deals with the diet plan, but exercise as well, since its main principle says "heal/cure yourself through proper diet and exercise".

The *Ayurvedic* system has different diet plans for diabetic patients. Foods that possess astringent or bitter taste help in reducing diabetic effect. *Jamun* (Eugenia jambolana) seeds *churna* (powder) is very effective in diabetes treatment because of the presence of antidiabetic factors

Our ancestors gave deep thought to the food culture. Indian culinary science propounded all the information thousands of years ago, the kind of information that modern culinary science tells us today...

Our forefathers had written a few thousand years ago that "diet and body, diet and mind, diet and attitude of mind are related to each other". This was indeed amazing. The holy book – *Bhagavad Gita* is estimated to be at anywhere between 5,000 – 6,000 years old. In the 17th *adhyaya* (chapter) of the *Gita*, shlokas 8, 9 and 10 explain the results that appear due to our diet on our life...

Persons having three types of nature – *sattvik*, *rajasic* and *tamsic* show the tendency to consume three types of foods and people's deeds depend on the three mental attitudes of a person.

ब्रह्मार्पणं ब्रह्म हविर्ब्रह्माग्नौ ब्रह्मणा हुतम् ।

ब्रह्मैव तेन गन्तव्यं ब्रह्मकर्मसमाधिना ॥

brahmārpaṇaṁ brahma havir brahmāgnau brahmaṇā hutam

brahmaiva tena gantavyaṁ brahma-karma-samādhinā

- *Lord Krishna, Gita*

Chapter 4 Shloka 24

ॐ सह नाववतु । सह नौ भुनक्तु । सह वीर्यं करवावहै ।

तेजस्वि नावधीतमस्तु मा विद्विषावहै ।

ॐ शान्तिः शान्तिः शान्तिः ॥

oṁ saha nāvavatu. saha nau bhunaktu. saha vīryaṁ karavāvahai.

tejasvi nāvadhītamastu mā vidviṣāvahai.

oṃ śāntiḥ śāntiḥ śāntiḥ

> *- Shanti Mantra from the Upanishads*

We are bearers of a perfect, scientific and nourishing ancient food culture and it is only pragmatic to take pride in this culture.

When did the chaos begin?

Jyotishavidya indicators mention damage to the body image, that which generates health disorders (bulimia, anorexia nervosa), is traceable to *Shani* and *Rahu*, in combinations with *Shukra* and *Chandra*. These correlate to the chaos that began as early in Vedic astrology or *Jyotiṣa*, which originated in ancient India around 2500 years ago.

Diet culture can be traced back to as early as Ancient Greek times, where moderation and regulation of food intake was promoted to attain "calmness". It was also represented as a marker of supreme self-control – one of the highest virtues in ancient Greece.

The first actual diet book came out in 1558 and is still in print. Luigi Cornaro was an extremely overweight Italian who had an epiphany when he was around 40 years old.

The first well-liked eating plan was called "Banting" named after William Banting. He described the specific low-carb, low-calorie diet that caused his significant weight loss in his 1863 booklet, Letter on Corpulence, addressed to the public.

The 1930s diet fads

The Beverly Hills, Acid Ash, Body Ph, and Alkaline Diets are just a few of the modern diets that were inspired by the most intriguing diets of the time. All foods were categorized into three groups by Dr. William Hay in 1935: alkaline, acidic, and neutral. Starches and carbohydrates are alkaline, whereas meats and other proteins are acidic, and the other substances are neutral. Combining acid and alkaline results in incomplete digestion, which is why you shouldn't do it. Henry Ford, the creator of automobiles, and Man Ray were two of Dr. Hay's many admirers. Despite persisting today, his arguments lack any basis in science.

In the 1930s, the Hollywood Grapefruit Diet was also published. This diet, which was an inspiration for the Scarsdale and other similar ones in the 1970s, consists of a half grapefruit, an egg, and one Melba toast for breakfast, six slices of cucumber for lunch, and a half grapefruit, two eggs, lettuce, and one tomato slice for supper. Another fad diet from the 1930s calls for only bananas and skim milk as food.

In his book "Slimming for the Million", Dr. Eustace Chesser advised overweight individuals to stay away from "fat-forming foods" and have meat, vegetables, and fruit for lunch and supper in addition to eggs and bacon for breakfast. Scientists and other professionals were making derogatory comments about obese individuals in the meantime. In a 1935 article, Professor Charles Lambie asserted that obesity was at its most prevalent.

Because of their peculiar look and inherent lack of respect, the Hollywood Diet and the Lemonade Diet, often referred to as the Master Cleanse and the Grapefruit Diet, respectively, were still popular. You only need to ingest one teaspoon each of cayenne pepper, lemon juice, and maple syrup in a glass of water six to twelve times daily for three days. Sylvia, a celebrity nutritionist, catered to movie stars, providing them with starvation diets and "fat-reducing" massages. In 1942, Metropolitan Life produced the first age and weight charts that showed the "ideal" weights for men and women based on their height.

Women's "plus-size" apparel was first made available by Sears Roebuck and Montgomery Ward in the middle of the 1940s. The notation was a regular size followed by a plus sign, for example, Size 14+.

To further study the origins, effects, prevention, and treatments of obesity, doctors established the National Obesity Society in 1949.

Two sets of participants in a 1950 British research study over-ate for a whole week. When thin people eat more food to burn off the extra calories, their metabolisms speed up. The researchers came to the conclusion that diet advice is cruel and outdated because the number of overweight people has not increased.

33% of people were overweight and 10% were clinically obese between 1950 and 1960. By 1969, 15% of individuals were fat, and 35% of adults were overweight. Nevertheless, until the Atkins movement in 1972, low-calorie, low-fat, and "diet" meals were still popular. Medical professionals also offered assistance to dieters in the form of prescription "diet pills", which contained amphetamines and dinitrophenol to speed up metabolism. These medications had been misused extensively for decades and were already often given for depression. Amphetamines were prescribed 8% of the time by "diet physicians" in "diet clinics" by the year 1970. According to Dr. Nicholas Rasmussen's estimate published in the journal Public Health, six to ten billion 10-mg pills were marketed.

Dietary supplements were still widely used. Dexatrim was first introduced in 1977, but the FDA removed it from sale in 2000 due to a connection to strokes. "Dr. Atkins' Diet Revolution" was published by Dr. Roger Atkins in 1972. His theories brought about a revolution in the diet business; hence, the title was not an error. In 1974, Dr. Atkins continued to develop a diet which used a variety of weight-loss meals in conjunction with the diet. At its peak, one in every eleven Americans followed the Atkins diet. In 1974, the American Psychiatric Association classified anorexia and bulimia as psychiatric illnesses that affect children and adolescents. The 1981 Beverly Hills Diet begins on a low-fat with 10 days of only eating fruit in a certain order. Three ears of corn on the cob, two tablespoons of butter, and bread are added on Days 11 through 18. Meat is not included until Day 19. Linda Grey and Liza Minnelli were two famous people who visited Beverly Hills. On November 15, 1988, Oprah Winfrey displayed her weight loss from a liquid protein fast on her TV program by pulling a wagon loaded with 67 pounds of fat across the stage. This was arguably the most spectacular diet-related event of the decade. She was wearing size 10 pants, but after starting to consume actual food again the next week, she claimed that they no longer fit. Refusing to eat, or anorexia, became popular in the media. In a 1985 Gallup survey, 9% of teenage females admitted to engaging in certain anorexic behaviors.

Gloria Stein, a pioneering feminist, said that eating disorders were caused by "gender prisons" and that they claimed 150,000 women's lives each year. In 1983, 101 deaths were really reported on death certificates.

To replace the outdated map of important food categories, the US government created the "food pyramid" in 1992.

Bread, grains, and cereal were at the bottom of the pyramid, with recommendations to consume 8 to 11 servings daily. Fruit and vegetables were next, with recommendations to consume 2-4 servings of fruit and 3-4 servings of vegetables per day. Dairy and meat were suggested to consume 2 to 3 servings per day. The recommendation was to "eat sparingly", with the focus being on fats and oils. The Food Pyramid is occasionally cited as some of the worst advice ever offered by those who do better on low-carb diets. Dr. Atkins' Diet Revolution was published in the 1970s, however Atkins Diet had resurfaced in the 1992 when it reached its height of popularity.

Anorexia and bulimia were recognized by the American Psychiatric Association in 1994, and "eating disorder not defined" was added to their list of mental diseases in 2013. The American Medical Association declared obesity an illness in 2013. This made it possible for some insurance companies, including Medicare, to cover the cost of bariatric procedures such placing a gastric band to reduce the size of the stomach, surgically removing a portion of the stomach.

In 2013, more than 179,000 of these operations were performed, an increase from 103,000 in 2003. In 2013, the American Psychiatric Association modified its definition of an eating disorder by removing "eating disorder undefined", but preserving anorexia and bulimia. "Cash incentives for weight loss" were another internet trend of the 2000s. You pay to join, then monthly after that, and if you lose weight, you get paid. Nowadays, millions of entries for items with complete nutritional information are available on new websites for dieters. One can even search through thousands of precise restaurant menu options.

The Baby Food Diet, the Clean Diet, Karl Lagerfeld, Paleo Diet, Five-Bite, Werewolf, Alkaline, Cotton Ball and KE are just a few of the fad diets that have been popular in the 2010s.

It is what it says it is: the baby food diet. Madonna and Demi Moore both attempted the Werewolf Diet, which causes you to fast according to the phases of the moon. You consume cotton balls as filler when following the cotton ball diet, which 1950s models formerly followed. One of the most bizarre diets is KE, which involves having food pumped into your body through feeding tubes rather than eating it.

Three things are likely to shape diets in the future:

Nutrigenomics, prescription medications, and more government control over the food supply.

Where are we today? The Indian market for health food is predicted to reach $30 million in five years on the back of rising demand for nutritious snacks, sweets and groceries. 2021 reports on the other hand that Americans could be giving up on diets. Like only 20% of persons were dieting in 2013, less than 16.5% in 2022, compared to 31% in 1991. Among Americans, just 23% stated they thought losing a specific amount of weight would make them more beautiful.

The medical profession is debating whether it is appropriate to recommend dieting to overweight patients given that the long-term success rates are fewer than 5%. All of them assume skinny individuals are healthy, but if someone loses weight, they will always require less calories and more activity, who is to say how their actions are affecting their metabolism? We are still a long way from deriving any conclusion for the same.

A person's eating habits are generally referred to as their "diet". The energy and nutrients you require for better health, illness management, and disease prevention are found in food.

The entire amount of food that a person consumes constitutes their diet. Despite the adaptability of humanity, each culture and/or person has certain culinary preferences or taboos. This can be due to ethical considerations or individual choices. An individual's dietary decisions may be more or less healthy.

Complete nutrition requires the consumption and absorption of vitamins, minerals, necessary amino acids from protein, vital fatty acids from fat-containing meals, as well as dietary energy in the form of carbs, protein, and fat.

Dietary habits and choices have a big impact on longevity, health, and quality of life. Natural, unprocessed foods are preferred to pre-packaged meals and snacks in a healthy diet. It is considered balanced such that it gives your body the vitamins, minerals, and other nutrients it requires to operate at its peak. It prioritizes plant-based foods above animal-based meals, particularly fruits and vegetables. There is a lot of protein in it. Salt and sugar content are minimal. It uses "good fats" and other nutrients from plants.

Exclusionary diets are ones that omit specific food categories or dietary groups for medical or personal reasons. Many people abstain from eating food produced from animals to varied degrees for health reasons, moral concerns, or to lessen personal environmental impact (flexitarianism, pescetarianism, vegetarianism and veganism).

Although we observed some individuals may need to take extra care to acquire enough protein, iron, calcium, zinc, and vitamin B12, most people may get enough nourishment from a balanced vegetarian or vegan diet.

Education, affluence, accessibility in the local area, and mental health have significant influences on food decisions. The kind of meals that are permitted are limited by some cultures and faiths.

Mediterranean, gluten-free, low-calorie, and low-FODMAP diets are a few examples of popular diets approach specific conditions. Every diet has its own specific set of guidelines that outline what is and isn't permitted. For instance, vegan diets don't include any animal products of any kind and exclusively include plant-based cuisine.

There is no "one-size-fits-all" diet or nutrition plan that works for everyone.

2. This & That Diet

"It's smarter to look at portions than to count calories."

- *Preetha Kkiran*

Fasting

"Intermittent fasting", a sort of fasting, prevents eating between particular times of the day. There are several variations of intermittent fasting, such as the 5:2 diet, alternate-day fasting, and time-restricted eating. Intermittent fasters eat all of their meals inside a specific time window, which unites all varieties.

Because it emphasises meals that are low in density and rich in water, a volumetric diet provides you the opportunity to select the things you want to eat (Calorie counting is not necessary).

This diet may potentially provide extra health benefits aside from weight loss. The volumetric diet is centred around foods that are abundant in fibre, antioxidants, vitamins, and minerals. A decreased risk of heart disease and various cancers, including colon cancer, has been linked to diets high in fibre.

The flexitarian diet is as flexible as they come, so if you're looking for a meal you can bring to buffets, gatherings, and athletic occasions, this one could be for you. You can reduce your carbon footprint and spend less money by consuming fewer animal products.

A diet high in meat tends to be more expensive and unfriendly to the environment than a flexitarian one. In addition to its positive effects on the social and environmental spheres, a flexible vegetarian diet provides a number of health benefits. Increased longevity and a lower incidence of diseases including diabetes, cancer, high cholesterol, and heart disease are two possible benefits of a flexible diet.

The hormone reset diet is a brief weight-loss plan that does not follow USDA recommendations and is not regarded as healthy. It claims to aid in your 6 to 7 kgs weight loss in just 21 days, however, any weight lost will probably be gained again. The majority of individuals would feel hungry after eating it since it has too few calories. Successful long-term weight loss depends on a balanced diet and frequent exercise.

Mediterranean food

The widely regarded cuisine is inspired by the eating and living habits of people who live in the Mediterranean, such as Greek communities.

A range of foods, social engagement, physical activity, and a wide variety of nutrients are all encouraged by the long-term lifestyle plan. The Mediterranean diet must include whole grains, vegetables, and lean protein sources like fish, legumes, and nuts, as well as healthy fats like olive oil. A Mediterranean diet may reduce your risk of acquiring diabetes, cancer, and heart disease, "U.S. News & World Report" consistently names it as the best overall diet.

People with inflammatory disorders or chronic inflammation may find an anti-inflammatory diet attractive. It emphasizes consuming nutrients that reduce physiological inflammation, such as fruits and vegetables. Alcohol and foods that induce inflammation, such processed foods, should be avoided.

The DASH diet aims to lower blood pressure and control it. The National Heart, Lung, and Blood Institute advises against eating foods that are high in sugar, fat, and salt.

On the other side, the DASH diet places a strong emphasis on fish, poultry, fruits, vegetables, whole grains, nuts, and low-fat dairy products.

Beware of Fad diets

The keto diet was initially used to treat epilepsy and advocates for consuming a lot of fat and very little carbs. It promises significant weight reduction by forcing the body into a state of ketosis, which occurs when there are not enough carbs for the body to use as fuel. It's important to keep in mind that no studies have been done to determine the long-term safety of the ketogenic diet.

The 3-Day Military Diet works well for short-term weight loss, but after you start a regular diet, you'll probably gain back any weight you lost while following the regimen.

Dr. Lulu Hunt Peters, who once weighed 199 kgs herself, was probably the first person to count calories and advise others to do the same. Her 1918 book, "Dieting and Health: With a Key to the Calories", sold over two million copies in 55 editions. Declaring that "being fat is sinful, and self-control is the key to slimness", Dr. Peters suggested a diet of 1200 calories a day for women to be eaten in 100-calorie units.

Nutritionists seldom advise these diets and even so, only when they are required to achieve specific nutritional or health objectives. When following these diet plans, it is likely that most of the weight you lose is in the form of water and lean muscle, and not body fat.

A healthy, balanced diet should consist of a mix of vegetables, fruits, grains, lean meats, beans, legumes, nuts, seeds, dairy products, and oils, according to the U.S. Department of Agriculture's (USDA) dietary standards. Additionally, the USDA specifies daily calorie estimates for women (1600 to 2200 calories) and adult males (2200 to 3000 calories).

Consider various eating strategies while keeping in mind your individual demands and dietary preferences, as there is **"no one diet that is effective for everyone"**.

Understanding the principles of healthy nutrition and how food fuels your body will help you make more informed decisions and create meals that nourish your body. Healthy nutrition is the cornerstone of good health.

To control their weight and health, many individuals count calories or rely on the number on a scale, but in recent years there has been a major backlash against this diet culture approach.

One approach is to retain weight reduction as a long-term goal, while the other is to completely reject the diet mentality and set objectives for health, wellbeing, and self-care instead. This catalysed the inception of this book ***Ditch the Diet; Dare to Define***.

The best plan is to skip weight loss as your motivational goal and practice self-care such as making peace with food, enjoying nourishing meals while respecting your appetite, and practicing meaningful exercise without trying to burn off the calories.

If you need help getting started, read on and get a wide array of solutions to improving almost every problem, including being more productive, achieving success, building stronger relationships, finding happiness, and maintaining good health.

Focus on slowing down, encouraging mindfulness, and tailoring your goals to where you are now to get where you want to be.

Weight Cycling

Yo-Yo dieting, also known as weight cycling, is the pattern of losing and regaining weight over and over again, so your weight is constantly fluctuating. While people generally think of weight loss as healthy, Yo-Yo dieting can actually damage your health, leading to heart disease, high blood pressure, and a higher BMI over time.

Yo-Yo dieting may occur in anybody, but it is especially common in people who struggle with their connection with food and their body image.

Typically, new diets claim that their plan will help you look and feel your best, which can entice someone who believes that losing weight would improve their life.

Dieting might sound like a beneficial thing to do for your health when society focuses so much attention on a person's weight or BMI (Body

Mass Index). While maintaining a healthy weight for your age, gender, and body type is essential, it is equally important how you get there.

Unfortunately, several popular diets promoted on social media are not sustainable or are extremely restricted, leading to Yo-Yo dieting since they cannot be maintained long-term. When this occurs regularly, it might have some harmful repercussions.

Yo-Yo dieting can have a variety of detrimental effects, such as reduced nutrient and hypocaloric intake, reduced thyroid function, reduced stamina, increased fatigue, and mood changes.

Weight reduction frequently results in a slowdown of the Resting Metabolic Rate (RMR). The term "adaptive thermogenesis" or "metabolic adaptation" may be used to describe this phenomenon. People should be aware of their food consumption, up their physical activity levels, and practice self-kindness in order to counteract chronic metabolic adaptation. They should also follow up with professionals who can provide them with a more personalized approach based on their particular circumstances and requirements.

Yo-Yo dieting may encourage the buildup of visceral fat in the stomach.

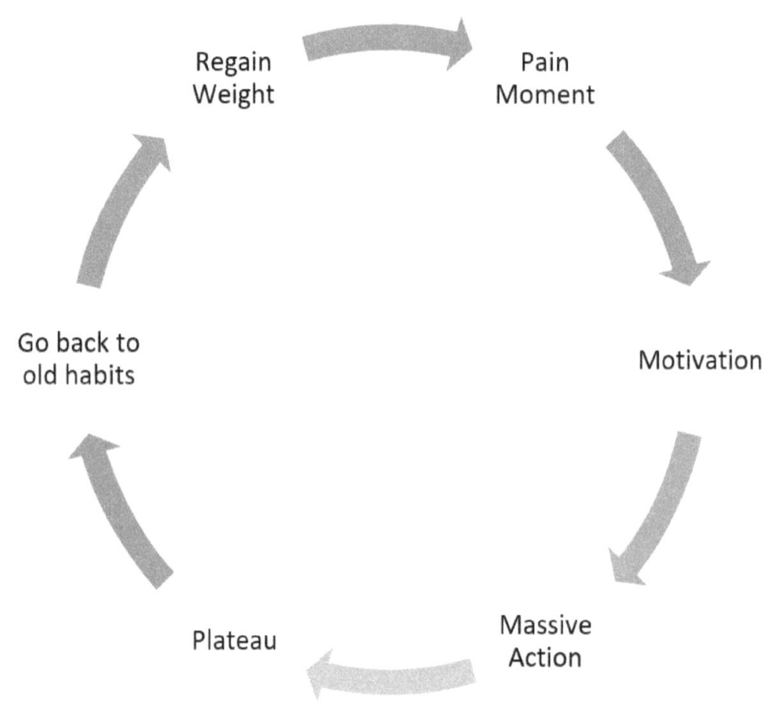

Yo-Yo Diet Cycle

Yo-Yo dieting raises the risk of developing an eating disorder and also takes some of the enjoyment out of eating. Having a long-term unhealthy and unbalanced relationship with food can cause disordered eating and possibly increase the chance of developing eating disorders like anorexia or bulimia.

3. Where does "I am on a DIET" start?

- *Preetha Kkiran*

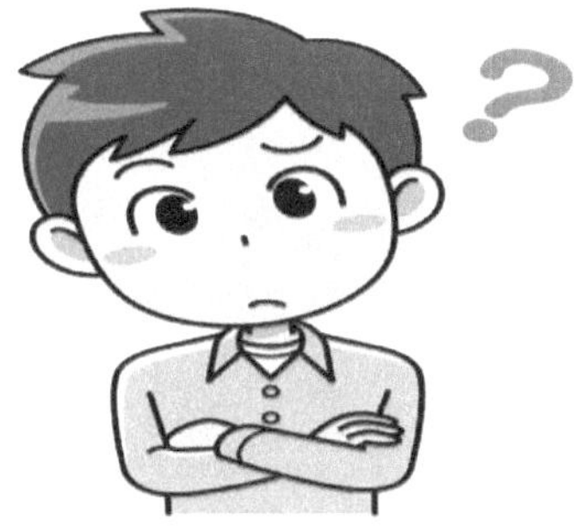

To reduce, maintain, or gain body weight, or to prevent and cure disorders like diabetes and obesity, dieting is the practice of eating food in a controlled manner. It has been demonstrated that different calorie-reduced diets, such as those prioritizing different macronutrients (low-fat, low-carbohydrate and such), aren't any more successful than another because weight reduction relies on calorie intake.

Long-term commitment to a diet is the strongest indicator of effectiveness because weight regain is common. The results of a diet, however, might vary greatly depending on the person.

For those individuals with weight-related health issues, some recommendations call for diets to reduce weight, but not for those who are otherwise healthy.

According to a poll, over half of all Indians, including 66.7% of those who are obese and 26.5% of those who are normal weight or underweight, try to reduce weight by dieting. Dieters with a higher death risk may include those who are overweight (but not obese), normal weight, or underweight, all of which are detrimental.

4. What is the right DIET approach?

"Those who mind don't matter and those who matter don't mind."

-   Preetha Kkiran

Chronic dieters frequently describe feelings of guilt and self-blame, irritation, anxiety, and sadness, as well as fatigue and attention problems. They always feel like failures because they keep "messing up my diet again", which makes them feel like they have no control over what they eat and lowers their self-esteem.

Make sure to include a variety of fruits, vegetables, whole grains, seeds, and nuts in your diet, along with foods high in protein like meat, fish, tofu, beans, and lentils, avocados, vegetable oils, and fatty seafood, as well as dairy products with low or no fat content like yogurt and cheese and soy products with added calcium.

There is still a place for certain salty and sweet pleasures like chips and chocolate ice cream, even though the aforementioned foods should make up the majority of what we eat during the day.

Do not categorize items as "good" or "bad" or eliminate entire food groupings from your daily intake.

As long as it is well-planned and contains a range of foods from all the food groups, such as whole grains, fruits, vegetables, beans, nuts, and seeds, as well as fat-free or low-fat dairy products or fortified soy versions, a vegetarian eating style can be a part of a healthy eating plan.

Due to diet culture's pervasiveness in all facets of society, it is impossible to completely escape it, but there are ways to both limit your exposure to it and speak out against it. *Ayurveda* deals with medicine, sciences and traditional dietary methods. It accommodates prosperity of wisdom on health and wellness sciences and is considered as *Upaveda* of *Atharveda*. 1200–900 BCE is when dieting person's references were recorded. We have been in the cycle for too long, however, this is the right time to start changing your diet and ditching the diet and defining yourself.

Avoid using any social media platforms, forums, online communities, or programming that encourages you to believe that you are not good enough as you are.

Media consumption has been shown to intensify negative self-evaluations, which is a fundamental aspect of diet culture.

It is hazardous to set a weight reduction target that is based on what a social media influencer, diet marketing, or Fad Diet book promises to be achievable.

Without professionalism, false statements and deceptions are frequent.

The bulk of overexcited theories lack solid scientific foundations. According to a meta-analysis of obesity treatments, the research subjects had actually regained more than 80% of the weight they had lost after 5 years.

The fact is that when someone follows unrealistic diets and sets themselves up for failure, they feel terrible about it.

On the other side, excessive scrolling can exacerbate mental health issues like melancholy and anxiety by triggering feelings of insecurity or FOMO (Fear of Missing Out).

A moderate middle ground is probably preferable for most of us when it comes to using social media. Setting certain boundaries may be necessary in order to find your own personal equilibrium.

Try using an app that lets you establish your daily time restrictions for social media or set up one day each week to take a break from it for better alternative social consumption. Then, use the free time you have to engage in positive things like reading a motivational book, practicing meditation, or even calling a friend for a real-world chat.

Take advantage of

"CAMPAIGN AGAINST NUTRITION QUACKS AND COURSES"

A great initiative by the Indian Dietetics Association to curb this misleading information for the safety of individual's battling health issues.

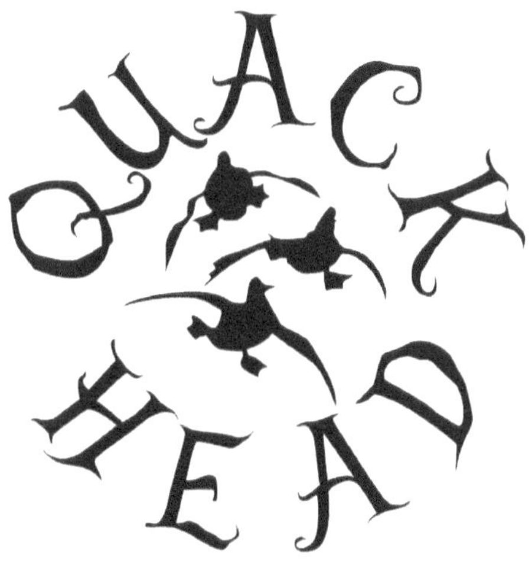

Try to be body-neutral

The concept of "body neutrality" holds that you should concentrate on what your body is capable of doing right now rather than what you would like it to look like.

It diverts your attention from attempting to alter or manage how you appear. Instead, it alters your perspective such that you have ambivalence about how you appear and are honoring what you can accomplish right now.

Body neutrality practices can assist you in letting go of diet culture and food labeling and working towards respecting your body in its current state.

Let us learn about our health through this ***Ditch the Diet*** book to gain a greater understanding of how focusing just on thinness and food restriction can be harmful to your health by reading and educating yourself about what total health is.

Additionally, this will aid in your comprehension of the several approaches to good health, including various body types and dietary habits.

Diet culture sometimes seems like an inevitable strain that everyone must endure. It's crucial to understand that dieting is not the only method to achieve health and that being slim does not imply health. Read on so that we can assist you if you are battling with disordered eating, an eating disorder, or are worried about your health, body image, or eating habits.

NutritionOnUrPlate and I, Preetha Kiran, have been striving hard all along my professional life and it is my endeavour through this book to reduce the stigma associated with being overweight, enhance inclusion, and change how society talks about weight reduction.

5. Who am I? (Body Image) Part 1

"Be proud of who you are and don't change for anyone."

-   Preetha Kkiran

India's National Institute of Health says that there is a need for the development of culturally sensitive instruments for diagnosis as well as for generating locally relevant epidemiological data about eating disorders from community and hospital settings. The cultural differences between East and West have contributed to variations in the presentation as well as challenges in the diagnosis.

पथ्ये सति गदार्तस्य किमौषधिनिषेवणैः ।

पथ्येऽसति गदार्तस्य किमौषधिनिषेवणैः ॥

Pathye sati gadārtasya bheṣajagrahaṇena kim

Pathye asati gadārtasya bheṣajagrahaṇena kim

"When diet is wrong, medicine is of no use;

when diet is correct, medicine is of no need."

-   Lolimbiraj, Vaidya Jivanam
Chapter 1 Verse 10

Referring to the National Eating Disorder Association (NEDA), which defines body image as how a person sees themselves, either when they see their reflection in the mirror or how they picture themselves mentally, it extends to how a person remembers, assumes, or generalizes their appearance, as well as their personal feelings towards their weight, height, and figure.

Body image may or may not relate to how a person actually appears but rather to their emotional attitudes, beliefs, and perceptions of their own body. Body image can range between positive and negative and may cause a person to feel different depending on the scenario or period in their life - either entirely positive, entirely negative, or a combination of both. Image concerns related to weight or other dimensions of appearance are now prevalent on a global scale. Given these high rates and the negative effects of body image concerns across society, it is important to increase our efforts to prevent and mitigate them.

We garner our own body image from a myriad of sources – the media, our peers, our parents, and our healthcare providers.

Cultural and social networks are powerful in how we develop body image ideals - many of which are thin standards of beauty that are unrealistic for people who are genetically larger to attain. Body size and shape can change predictably and normally with age, yet the societal pressure that many individuals face to change their bodies is fairly high.

Dissatisfaction with one's body is starting at an earlier age than ever before, even prior to adolescence, which highlights the very real necessity of the need for body-positive discussions and interventions from a young age.

If you have a negative body image, it means that the majority of your thoughts and perceptions about your own physical appearance are negative. This is often seen in the form of a young teenager or a middle-aged adult catching a glimpse of themselves in the mirror or shop window and wishing that they looked different from their reflection.

Negative body image can result from brief and unpredictable moments like these, heightened anxiety in social situations, or a constant negative internal dialogue about your body that stays with you for most of the day.

A distorted body image can also lead to negative feelings about your body because you do not have a realistic view of your appearance.

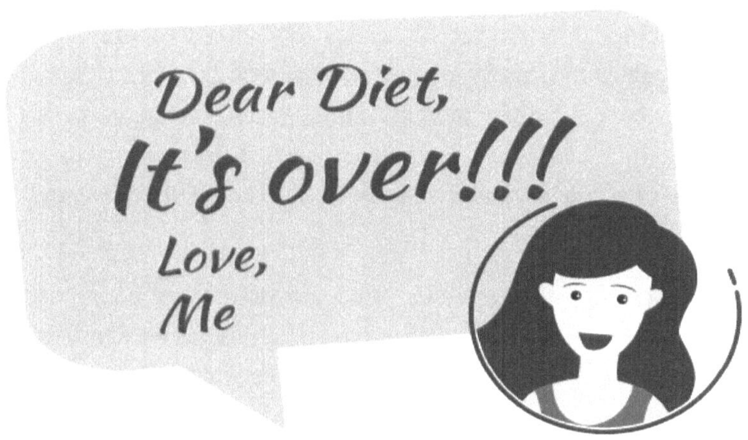

What exactly is positive body image?

Positive body image, on the other hand, is when a person has self-confidence, self-pride, and body positivity about their physical appearance.

People who accept their bodies have a strong sense of worthiness, attractiveness, and strengths that are not tied to their outward appearance, The term "body acceptance" is frequently used because it promotes respecting your body and treating it with kindness even if you don't feel particularly good about it.

Being body-positive, or having body acceptance, encourages considerably more than simply personal approval of one's own body; it also extends to other aspects of a person's life, such as their behaviours and mental health, love relationships, professional performance, and financial position.

When you have a positive body image, you are more likely to have confidence and be willing to try new things and take risks because the thought of your body getting in the way of your dreams is much less of a concern. You can see beyond your physical body and value yourself as a human being, and you are more likely to treat others with respect, love, care, and kindness.

Body checking is the process of analyzing your body through numerous methods such as looking in the mirror, weighing yourself, or touching or pinching yourself. While there is nothing fundamentally wrong with examining your body once in a while, when it influences how you feel about yourself or becomes impulsive, it can lead to psychological problems.

Body checkers may concentrate on certain portions of their bodies that they detest or begin to compare their bodies to those of others. Some people check their bodies hundreds of times each day, which can have an impact on their mental health and quality of life. It is critical to recognize the indicators of body-checking and get expert assistance.

Body Checking can affect your **Quality of Life** and may become an obsessive cycle of physically inspecting your body and then having obsessive and negative thoughts about your body. Body Checking has been demonstrated to cause body dissatisfaction regardless of whether a body area is examined. Furthermore, body checking might alter your mood and make you more self-conscious about your body weight and appearance.

Body Checking keeps us preoccupied with our bodies and reinforces the idea that the shape and size of our bodies are the most important things about us; Body Checking frequently begins as a means to reduce worry. We believe that checking will help us feel better, but most of the time, it leads to negative thoughts about our body and thus ourselves.

The relaxation that may occur from Body Checking is rarely lasting, and the need to check returns along with the uneasiness. This consumes more and more of our mental space and energy and can have a significant impact on our mental health.

While Body Checking can be a problem regardless of eating habits, research suggests that the two are frequently linked. Body Checking, particularly restriction, can be used to sustain disordered eating patterns.

Body Checking is frequently observed in the context of eating disorders, disordered eating, and unhappiness with one's body image. We address the entire spectrum of symptoms, not just the body.

Correcting body-checking behavior may also aid behaviour reduction of eating-problem symptoms.

It's vital to treat these behaviors, as they are connected to poor mental health, depression, a lower quality of life, and poor self-esteem.

Body Checking is a common obsessive behavior used to treat body-related anxiety. After eating, you could feel the urge to pinch yourself or check your reflection to see whether your physique has altered.

Every person who struggles with body checking is unique. Still, it may be beneficial to learn how to use **Mindfulness** to be able to identify the temptation to body check without acting on it.

Practicing mindfulness may be very beneficial for improving observation skills, being more cognizant of one's thoughts and desires, and creating room for intentional decisions as opposed to automatic ones.

Observing desires to body-check and gently exploring them without acting on them. You might find it useful to reflect on these issues:

- What comes to mind when the temptation to body-check strikes?

- What feelings come up?

- Does the strength of the cravings change as you investigate them?

Body Checking frequently develops into an obsession, which causes a host of detrimental mental health problems, such as decreased self-esteem and body image concerns. Body Checking is frequently linked to problematic eating patterns, which, if left untreated, can develop into serious eating disorder.

To address this habit, it is advisable to work with a licensed psychotherapist such as *NutritionOnUrPlate* who has expertise with body image concerns from a health- and size-informed perspective.

Body checkers are more likely to restrict their food intake and exhibit early signs of an eating disorder. Dietary restriction and frequent body checking are both symptoms of eating disorders and the fear of gaining weight, respectively.

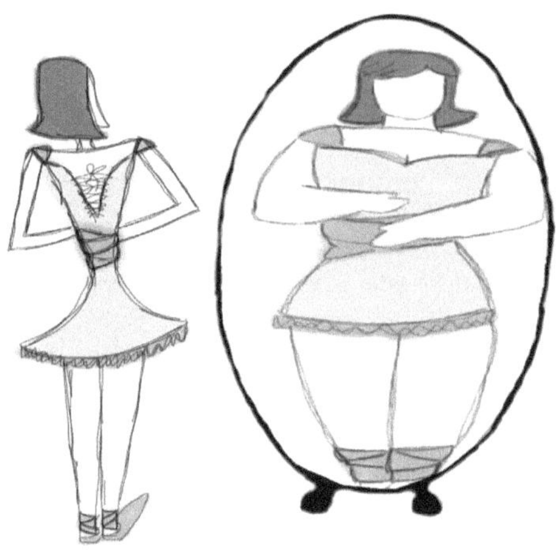

6. Where am I?
(Under/Ideal/Overweight) Part 2

"You are what you choose to become."

- *Preetha Kkiran*

The term "body composition" is used by us to describe the body's proportions of fat, water, bone, muscle, skin, and other lean tissues.

Understanding your body composition gives you more in-depth knowledge about your health. Due to differences in body composition, two people who weigh the same amount might have significantly different health and fitness requirements.

Body composition is significant since it gauges your level of fitness and general health by calculating your body fat percentage. Your bathroom scale is unable to distinguish between how much of your weight is made up of muscle and how much is fat. Evaluations of body composition might be more muscle and less fat often indicate a higher degree of performance.

Body fat includes all the stored fat in your body.

There are two types of body fat:

Subcutaneous fat: This is the layer of fat under your skin. It insulates and protects your body.

Visceral fat: This is the fat that surrounds and cushions your abdominal organs.

In addition to insulating and protecting your body, fat provides energy, carries fat-soluble vitamins, produces certain hormones, and serves as a building block for cell membranes.

You need a certain amount of body fat to perform these functions—this is known as essential fat.

Body fat percentage is the percent of fat that makes up your total body weight. Many factors influence your body fat percentage, including sex, age, fitness level, and lifestyle

Ideal body composition for both men and women

Men should have a somewhat lower body fat percentage than women. Age and gender have an impact on a person's body fat percentage. Adiposity or fat accumulation as it is commonly known, rises with age in both men and women. According to studies, estrogen, which is only found in females, controls how much fat is stored. Improved nursing, fetal growth, and fertility are all benefits of effective fat storage.

A Tabular look at Body Fat Norms

Athletes tend to have a lower body fat percentage than people who are physically fit because having less fat improves their athletic performance. However, when body fat percentages dip too low, athletic performance suffers, and immune function declines. On the flip side, a very high body fat percentage is a risk factor for chronic illnesses like diabetes, high blood pressure, and heart disease.

Body Fat Percent Norms for Men and Women

Description	Women	Men
Essential Fat	10% to 13%	2% to 5%
Athletes	14% to 20%	6% to 13%
Fitness	21% to 24%	14% to 17%
Acceptable	25% to 31%	18% to 24%
Obese	Over 32%	Over 25%

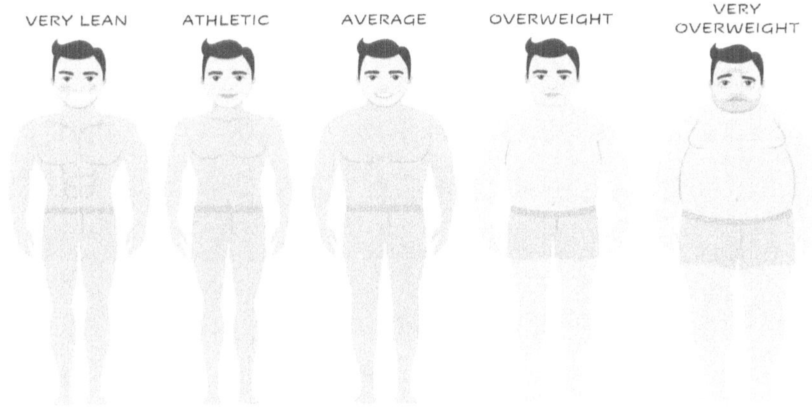

Body Composition vs. Body Mass Index:

Body composition and body mass index (**BMI**) are tools that assess body fatness. However, the methods used to measure body composition and BMI differ. Additionally, BMI may not provide accurate results in all situations.

Body Mass Index (BMI) is a dated, biased measure that doesn't account for several factors, such as body composition, ethnicity, race, gender, and age. Despite being a flawed measure, BMI is widely used today in the medical community because it is an inexpensive and quick method for analyzing potential health status and outcomes.

Body Mass Index

BMI is a tool that has been used by health professionals to assess body fatness and health. It's a mathematical equation that compares your weight to your height.

BMI = (weight in pounds) / (height squared) X 703

For example: (150 pounds) / (66 inches x 66 inches) X 703 = 24

This BMI table is from the Centers for Disease Control and Prevention (CDC).

- Less than 18.5 = underweight

- 18.5 to 24.9 = healthy weight

- 25.0 to 29.9 = overweight

- 30 or higher = obesity

You don't need any special equipment to measure BMI, making it a quick tool to assess body fat and health.

There are several ways to measure body composition. However, you need more than a bathroom scale and a calculator to figure out what percentage of your weight comes from fat and what percentage comes from muscle. *NutritionOnUrPlate* provides many of the tools that can determine the same so as to design your exclusive dietary approach towards good health.

7. Shasktrakum

(Tools to determine Body Type)

"It is not the tools we use that make us good, but rather how we employ them".

Bioelectrical Impedance

Bioelectrical Impedance (BIA) is a tool that estimates your body composition by measuring your body's resistance to a low-level electric current, or impedance. Muscles have a lower resistance to an electric current than fat.

Skinfold Measurements

Skinfold measurements involve the use of special callipers that measure the skinfold—subcutaneous fat—on different parts of your body. Fitness trainers use skinfold measurements to assess body fat because they're quick and convenient.

Body composition is a useful source of knowledge for body fat percentage. However, since your body form is specific to you, there are unavoidable aspects that might have an impact on your composition, such as …

Age: As you age, you lose muscle, which changes the makeup of your body. However, a decline in physical activity is the main cause of age-related muscle loss.

Genes: Your genetic makeup determines your body shape and composition, and depending on how much body fat you inherit, it can be more difficult for you to reduce.

Hormones: Hormones also affect how the body is made. The male sexual hormone testosterone makes muscles bigger.

Sex: Women have more body fat than men do as a result of heredity and hormones.

To change your body composition, you need the right balance of physical activity and nutrition to reach your goals. Slow and steady changes work best when you want to increase muscle and lose fat. It's important to remember that some factors will remain out of your control.

Before making any changes to your diet or workout routine, consult with your primary care provider or a registered dietitian for guidance.

Your body composition may help you better understand your current level of health and fitness. It can also serve as a measuring tool to monitor progress when starting a new fitness or wellness program.

When trying to change your physique to improve your fitness level, it is important to implement a safe and effective workout routine and a balanced eating plan.

What Does It Mean to Be Underweight?

Many healthcare professionals use mathematical equations like the Body Mass Index (BMI) as tools.

The BMI assesses your weight status by comparing your weight to your height. The calculation estimates body fatness, which health professionals use as a screening tool to determine disease risk. However, the BMI isn't meant to serve as a diagnostic tool for body fatness or a singular measure of overall health.

A BMI that falls between 18.5 and 24.9 is considered a normal or healthy weight range, while a BMI less than 18.5 falls within the underweight range.

The BMI is a dated and biased measuring tool for weight and health that doesn't account for several factors that influence both, such as body composition, ethnicity, race, gender, and age.

Despite being a flawed measure, BMI is widely used in the medical community because it's an inexpensive and quick method for analyzing potential health status and outcomes.

Measuring your body composition may provide a more accurate picture of your weight and health. Body composition compares how much of your total weight comes from lean body mass and how much is from fat. The percentage that comes from body fat is used to assess health.

- Healthy body fat percentage for men: 17.6 to 25.3%

- Healthy body fat percentage for women: 28.8 to 35.7%

Men with less than 17.6% body fat and women with less than 28.8% body fat are below normal weight, or underweight, according to a 2018 study published in the Journal of Exercise Rehabilitation. Fit individuals and athletes, however, may have lower body fat percentages and be at a healthy weight.

Underweight

The signs of undernutrition or underweight might be very different. Underweight individuals may have acute weariness, low blood pressure, and potentially even low blood sugar. They could also experience colds, nausea, and dizziness. Due to a deficiency in vitamins and minerals like magnesium and potassium, which are necessary for muscular contraction and relaxation, people may even have difficulties sleeping and develop cramps.

We frequently concentrate on the disadvantages connected with being overweight when discussing weight and the risk of health problems. However, being underweight may also be bad for your health.

You run the danger of developing multiple vitamin deficiencies, osteoporosis, a weakened immune system, and infertility, among other health issues.

Include vitamins and minerals

You cannot obtain enough nutrients and energy when you are underweight to maintain a healthy weight. This implies that you are unable to acquire a sufficient number of vitamins and minerals.

Being underweight increases your risk of vitamin deficiencies. Your body's ability to operate is impacted if critical nutrients are not present in sufficient amounts.

These dietary deficiencies might lead to health issues including anaemia from a lack of iron, folate, or vitamin B12; poor wound healing from a vitamin C deficiency; or night blindness from insufficient vitamin A consumption.

Osteoporosis

A dangerous bone disorder called osteoporosis results in porous, brittle bones that are more prone to breaking. One can have osteoporosis at any age. Eating poorly raises your risk.

You need an appropriate quantity of calcium and vitamin D to develop bone mass throughout childhood and preserve it as an adult. You probably aren't receiving enough calcium or vitamin D if you're underweight and not getting all the nutrients you need. In fact, our observations have shown that a lot of underweight people don't receive enough vitamin D.

Immune system dysfunction

Your immune system aids in the prevention of illnesses and infections. A balanced diet with an appropriate number of important nutrients needs to be consumed for optimum immune system behaviour. This remains true even as no single meal of supplement can improve immunological health.

You cannot obtain all the nutrients required for a good immune system if you are underweight because you are not eating enough. This can weaken your immune system and make you more susceptible to acquiring any cold going around your office.

Obstacles to Fertility

There is a link between low body fat and being underweight, and your body requires a particular quantity of fat to carry out its necessary duties. Although the majority of people believe that having too much fat is unhealthy, not having enough fat is also harmful.

Fertility issues may arise if you are underweight and have a low body fat percentage. Insufficient body fat has an impact on hormone synthesis, which impacts both male and female fertility.

How to Deal with Underweight

Consult your health care physician or a qualified nutritionist if you are underweight and seeking a way to gain weight. They can provide advice tailored to your particular needs and a precise assessment of your weight and any health effects.

Although eating has an impact on weight, there are other factors, such as heredity, physical activity, and medicine that have an impact on your body size.

For the treatment of undernutrition, modern paediatrics has recommended food control towards restoring the various deficiencies.

Despite the fact that being slim is frequently regarded as "ideal", there is a bias in favour of smaller people. As per our survey, many Indians believe that it is okay to say that someone is too thin and that they should eat more to put on weight. However, being overweight and being healthy are not synonymous.

You don't necessarily need to put on weight just because you're little or even underweight, according to the statistics. The presence of a healthy weight is not always "seen" as abnormal or indicative of an eating disorder.

How can I go from Under to Ideal?

Ayurveda suggests *Ahara Dosha* as the main predisposing factor, Disorder and *Alpasana* and *Vishamasana* (false habits of intake). Especially results in the development of *Karshya*.

Pharmacotherapies like *Bruhmana*, *Rasayana*, and *Vrisya* have been advocated in the classics for the management of *Karshya*.

In modern paediatrics, diet management and restoration of the different deficiencies have been advised for treatment of Undernutrition.

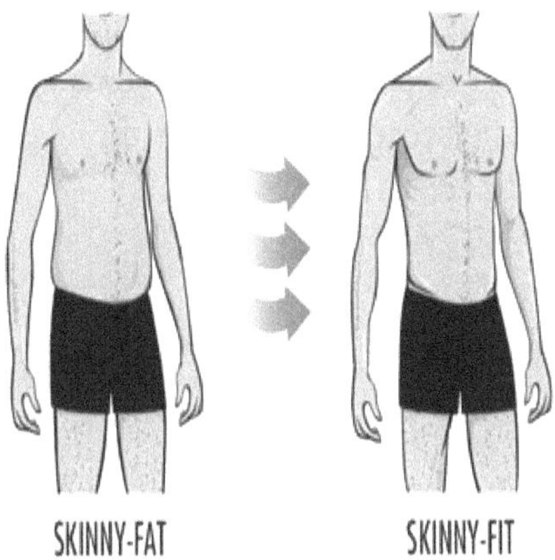

Gaining weight can be just as challenging for some people as losing it. While eating calorie-dense meals may make you gain a few pounds, they don't necessarily give your body the nourishment that it requires.

You must have a balanced diet that is rich in a range of nutrient-dense foods if you want to gain weight healthily.

1. Eating five to six small meals every day.

2. Drinking nutrient-rich drinks (milk, juice, smoothies) between meals.

3. Cheese, nuts, seeds, or dried fruit as a snack.

4. Salads and soups with shredded cheese, almonds, or beans as a garnish.

5. Adding nut butter to rotis, breads, pita, khubooz.

6. Adding dry milk powder to yogurt, cereal, or mashed potatoes.

7. Strength training may help improve muscle mass.

8. Make sure your diet has enough protein if you're working out to gain more muscle mass.

As I studied through the journals for compiling this book, I came across a recommendation in the British Journal of Sports Medicine that aiming for 0.7 grams of protein per pound of body weight when working out helps gain weight. Your weight isn't always the best indicator of health. A healthy weight varies from person to person and isn't something you can really "see". Being underweight because you're not eating enough affects your health now and in the future.

Skinny fat

A word frequently used to describe people who are "thin" yet have a high body fat percentage.

The medical term "normal weight obesity" refers to someone whose weight is "normal" for their height.

The majority of specialists concur that it could do more damage than benefit. "Skinny fat" turns the conversation away from the dangers of normal-weight obesity and onto looks, which is an unwelcome and counterproductive outcome of diet culture.

In many ways, the term "skinny fat" supports diet culture. Shaming someone based on their body weight, shape, size, or appearance is always detrimental.

What's more, this phrase is a form of weight stigma, and weight stigma – independent of weight itself – has been found to contribute to poorer health outcomes.

Unfortunately, our society makes it seem that as long as you look good, it's all that matters. The appearance of being skinny seems to outweigh being fit.

Individuals who are already struggling with eating disorders are hyper-focused on not only being "healthy", but they also tend to place additional value on the size of their bodies. The phrase skinny fat means that even though you are skinny, you are also fat. It makes the societal ideals that are already impossible to achieve even more unachievable. It is yet another way that diet culture can trigger more people and cause more damage.

No matter what your level of body fat is, maintaining a healthy weight, doing regular exercise, and growing muscle may all contribute to a longer and healthier life. Having a positive connection with food is also essential; when our bodies are optimally nourished and moving in a way that feels good for each of us individually, they thrive and function best.

You should consider how you feel about food and activity in addition to eating to meet your nutritional needs. A specific method of eating might not be the healthiest if it makes you feel guilty, embarrassed, or stressed.

If you're comparing yourself to this idea of "skinny fat", please realize that you don't need to change anything about yourself or your body based on what you hear in the media. Before adopting any health or eating related changes, pay attention to how you feel, listen to your body when it makes sense, and seek the opinion of a reliable specialist.

Exercise and Nutrition Are Vital for All Body Types

58% of studies revealed a relationship between a history of weight cycling and increasing weight around the stomach or belly. Unfortunately, **Visceral fat**, or fat that accumulates in the centre of the body, is linked to a variety of potentially fatal illnesses, including heart disease, stroke, and heart attacks. You may be predisposed to Type 2 Diabetes. While being overweight might raise your risk of diabetes in general, case-in-point, Yo-Yo dieting can have the reverse impact, even raising your chance of acquiring Type 2 Diabetes. A restricting or binge eating pattern, which is common in weight cycling, can lead to chronic blood glucose spikes that may increase the risk of Type 2 diabetes.

Muscle building is essential for strength, mobility, and healthy aging, but Yo-Yo dieting can undermine our body's muscle mass and current body fat.

When people talk about losing weight, what they want to do is change their body composition by losing fat by burning a few more calories than they consume while either maintaining or gaining muscle. If a person loses a pound of fat but gains a pound of muscle, their weight will remain constant, but their body composition will be healthier as their body fat percentage will be lower.

If you've relied on diets to lose weight for years or even decades, it might be difficult to break the pattern of Yo-Yo dieting.

NutritionOnUrPlate says it is critical to develop a long-term dietary approach.

8. Saptah Gyan Sutras (The Seven Secrets)

"There is nothing either good or bad, but thinking makes it so"

- *A quote from William Shakespeare's tragedy, Hamlet*

SUTRA 1

Small lifestyle changes can lead to big results for your health, so try these seven for a healthier you.

1. **Stop classifying foods as "good" or "bad".** Depending on how you think about food, you might be inclined to describe particular meals as "good" or "bad". However, doing so, may skew your perception of what is and isn't nutritious. When it comes to many of these items, it's often that the food itself is not the issue, but how much or how frequently we consume it. The problem is that making them off-limits gives them absolute power and removes your sense of self-control.

   I have done a thorough reference and study to conclude that a ***"No Diet"*** diet i.e., Intuitive Eating is the go-to Mantra as quoted by *Lord Krishna* in *Shrimad Bhagavad Gita*.

   "For him who is moderate in food and recreation, moderate in exertion in all actions, moderate in sleep and wakefulness, yoga destroys all pain and suffering (caused by birth and death)"

   Ditch the Diet; Dare to Define ruminates over these very same principles.

2. **Intuitive Eating** - an approach to eating that focuses on the body's response to cues of hunger and satisfaction, aiming to foster a

positive relationship with food as opposed to mere control over one's weight.

Dieting is the polar opposite of Intuitive Eating. Intuitive Eating entails paying attention to your body's natural signs, such as hunger and fullness, and any adverse effects that may occur when you ingest specific meals. Intuitive Eating habits boost health, including a lower incidence of Type 2 diabetes.

Intuitive Eating guides balanced and diverse food choices without restriction or deprivation by tuning into your body's unique and individual needs. Respecting our hunger and fullness cues, results in increased satisfaction and enjoyment as compared to Yo-Yo dieting.

3. **Self-care and stress management** should be prioritized. When we are stressed, we have less energy to devote towards living a healthy lifestyle. Incorporating self-care and working on stress reduction may assist and even improve our quality of life.

    When our metaphorical cup is empty and we're stressed, we generally turn to food for energy. A good stress management plan that includes stress-relieving activities like meditation, yoga, and journaling can actually serve as a Yo-Yo dieting avoidance strategy.

4. **Reach out to *NutritionOnUrPlate*** or a similar Medical and/or healthcare Professional. Seeking the assistance of a healthcare specialist, whether a registered dietitian or a mental health professional who specializes in disordered eating patterns may help you sketch a nutritious, balanced, and individualized meal plan for your needs. Getting to the root of your desire to lose weight and understanding the thoughts that drive food decisions can help break the weight-cycling phase.

5. **Practice Body neutrality**. This is similar to body positivity that focuses more on acceptance than self-love.

Weight neutrality, or "weight-neutral" movement, is an approach that aims to depart from the typical weight-centric focus on body weight and BMI and shift to improved lifestyle behaviours.

Weight neutrality aims to shift the emphasis from being weight-normative (using weight and weight loss when defining health) to bring more weight-inclusive (viewing health and wellness as multi-faceted)

6. **Talk to a near and dear one**.

Family and friends form a critical support system and you can always rely on their backing when something is new or challenging. Following this, it's usually helpful to seek advice from someone who has professional experience in this field.

7. **Consume Whole Grains**

Making your grains whole is a snappy slogan and a good, yet simple, improvement. Choose whole grains such as whole-wheat bread, pasta, red or brown rice, buckwheat, quinoa, oats, unpolished millets. The millets program, promoted by the *Poshan Abyaan* in India, to increase your fibre intake and lower your risk of cardiovascular disease and cancer, is gaining tremendous response.

You'd want to commit to trying one new grain/millet every month, delving into the fascinating realm of lesser-known grains like Sorghum (*jowar*), Amaranth (*rajgira*), Kamut, Pearl Millet (*bajra*), Finger Millet (*ragi*), Foxtail Millet (*kangni*), Barnyard Millet (*samwa*), Little Millet (*kutki*), Kodo Millet (*kodra*), Proso Millet (*chena*), Browntop Millet (*andua*) amongst others.

9. Satah Viddhi

(The Hexad game)

"Don't just sit around waiting for others, Just Do It!!!"

-   Preetha Kkiran

SUTRA 2

1. Start Walking

You might not be able to prepare for a marathon in the next 12 months, but you will be able to walk actively. Walking requires no extra equipment and is a simple form of exercise for the majority of individuals. A regular brisk walk can help you control your weight, lower your blood pressure, improve your bone health, and lower your risk of Type 2 diabetes, among other benefits.

If you are not currently walking at all or believe you could only accomplish one or two walks each week, it is still a realistic aim. The idea is to create reasonable and achievable objectives for yourself.

You can even go the extra mile, quite literally in this case, by finding a walking buddy. Having a partner provides built-in workout accountability, while social time spent with a friend will elevate your emotional well-being. Be sure to talk to a healthcare provider before beginning any type of rigorous exercise regime. *NutritionOnUrPlate* is always here to assist.

2. Eat More Fermented Foods

Eating more fermented foods may not be at the top of most people's goals. But before you turn up your nose at the prospect of a daily dose of sauerkraut, remember these multiple delicious options for fermented foods – all of which come with probiotics that promote gut health and reduce inflammation.

Upping your intake of foods like yogurt, or homemade *dahi*, pickle or *idlies*, kombucha, miso, and kimchi could yield meaningful results for your health.

3. Set a Consistent Bedtime

Putting children to bed on time is as good an idea as it is for adults. Adults, according to research, benefit by going to bed at the same hour every night. Referring to a 2018 study – a regular bedtime, rather than the overall amount of sleep, could be the key to many facets of improved health.

Clients at *NutritionOnUrPlate* have shown that going to bed at around the same time every night lowers the risk of obesity, cardiovascular disease, stress, and depression, particularly among older individuals.

4. Drink adequate water every day, every time

You've heard about the several benefits of being hydrated, which range from a brighter complexion to easier digestion to increased weight loss. There is no optimal goal for regular hydration since the "eight glasses a day" slogan is not universal. Constipation, headaches, tiredness, and dry/chapped lips are all signs that your body is not getting enough water. If any of these symptoms seem similar, it may be time to increase your fluid intake by drinking from a reusable, copper *Tamba* vessel/ water bottle every day.

5. Mix in your Salad Greens

Consider changing up your salad greens. If you usually include iceberg lettuce as the backbone of your salads, try a more nutrient-dense option like spinach, kale, or rocket.

These darker greens include more significant vitamins and minerals, including iron, vitamin K, potassium, and vitamin C. Once you've made the move and your tastes have adjusted to these richer-flavoured vegetables, you might find it easier to **Go Green**!

6. Concentrate on Nutritious Snacks

Overhauling your whole eating plan is time-consuming and often an overkill. Adding healthy snacks is a good way to start changing your nutritional habits. Each morning, include a piece of fruit, a hard-boiled egg, low-fat yogurt, or a traditional *chikki* /granola bar in your work or gym bag. This way, you'll have something nutritious for as between-meals snack. If you work from home, you may prepare and store these snacks ahead of time for a quick grab-and-go alternative when you're hungry.

While setting objectives, *NutritionOnUrPlate* advises you to keep in mind that everyone is at a different stage. These simple modifications are basic suggestions that have a huge positive impact.

Keep in mind to start small but start today. Going for a stroll outside once a week is preferable to not going at all. Similarly, a few more sips of water every day is a good place to start. Change can be difficult and intimidating, so start right now with goals you can manage and attain.

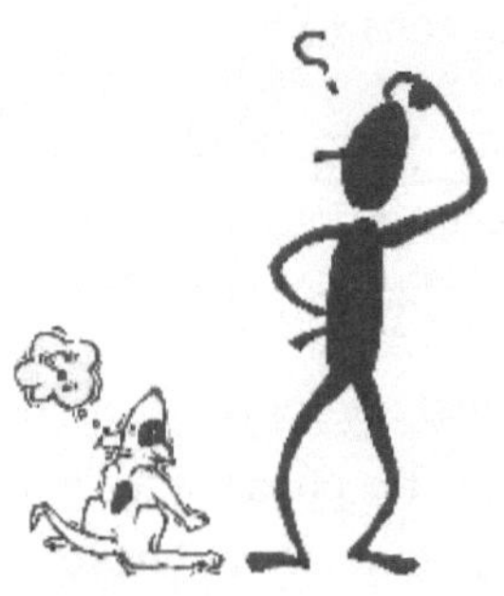

When it comes to nutrition facts and health benefits, understanding nutritional diversity helps you make smart choices for certain foods and beverages ranging from fruits, vegetables to whole grains.

Understanding what is going into your body has the ability to make all the difference in your personal welfare, whether your goal is weight control, heart health, diabetes management, or simply increasing general awareness.

Small, everyday decisions about your food, fitness, and overall well-being have the potential to change your life. However, this does not necessarily make them easy to maintain. Searching the internet, for diet or related workout subjects may be daunting, leading to a rabbit hole of phony fads and misleading promises.

10. Kayasamthosha

(I am what I am)

"Don't be afraid of who you are. Embrace who you are."

- *Preetha Kkiran*

Accepting your body, whether you are content with it or not, is "**body acceptance**".

Body image refers to all the ideas, perceptions, actions, and attitudes that you have about your body and appearance. It includes both positive and negative thoughts.

Being critical of your body in ways that affect your emotional and physical welfare might result in having a negative body image. These unfavourable thoughts may become dysfunctional for certain people and necessitate medical care.

Positivity about your body won't take over your thoughts and interfere with your happiness or general well-being if you learn to accept it.

Diet culture propagates the false notion that physical, psychological, and overall welfare are less important than having a **perfect body**. Diet culture normalizes the management of your body through nutrition by imposing dietary restrictions on what and how much you consume. Disturbed eating and disturbed body image may result from this.

Many people take longer than necessary to reach body acceptance. Working towards **body neutrality** may help you feel better if you have a particularly poor body image. Body neutrality is the grey area between embracing and rejecting your body at the same time.

Gender identity and other physical or mental characteristics may make it difficult for some people to accept their bodies.

Formulating a strategy to address some of these issues requires help and medical advice, and working with a therapist will definitely serve your needs better in this area.

Get on the wagon and read further if you're ready to practice **Body Acceptance**. It's not necessary to think of your body as something ideal, aesthetically pleasing, or that you shouldn't wish to alter it in any manner.

If you are prepared to accept your body as "good enough" by your own criteria, body acceptance is working for you.

It also indicates that you are aware that these criteria are distinct from the limited norms advocated by society regarding physical appearance, which lead to overall poor body frames.

"Unlearn years of dieting and unleash yourself."

\- *Preetha Kiran*

I am the best, indeed!

If you try to think positively about your body and reject negative ideas, that can be a definition of body acceptance.

Body positivity maintains a system in which beauty is prioritized.

Body acceptance emphasizes accepting your "flaws" and features of your physique that do not meet rigid societal standards.

The emphasis is still on physical attractiveness where flaunting and showcasing bodies on social media has become a norm of sorts.

Body acceptance is related to body neutrality; in that, it focuses on what your body can do rather than how it appears. Body acceptance is more complicated and entails realizing that you have aspects of your body that you are not content with and working on accepting these traits. Let our team at *NutritionOnUrPlate* assist you in achieving body acceptance.

Body acceptance is a personal journey that is unique to each individual. Although it may be preferable to go through it with a therapist, there are several "starting point" tactics that you may utilize to gain momentum through us.

Social media purge

Take stock of your abilities. Make a list of the things that you enjoy and your body can do for you right now. It might be your speed, distance running, or even fine motor abilities for handicraft.

Practice self-compassion

Try to counteract negative ideas with self-compassion. Forgive yourself and work on replacing negative ideas with positive ones. Instead of labelling your unpleasant feelings, consider watching them and seeing them as ephemeral, passing thoughts. Allow these ideas to "pass by" and then let them go. This might help you reinterpret and reframe your thoughts.

Body acceptance is a process that necessitates rejecting messages that you may have been exposed to for years as a result of media and cultural pressures.

It does not happen overnight, and it is not an all-or-nothing proposition. You can gradually progress towards body acceptance, beginning with body neutrality.

This transition is difficult, and ***Ditch the Diet; Dare to Define*** book is a valuable resource that provides a tailored, actionable guidance plan.

11. Kranti (The Revolution Begins)

Health at Every Size first appeared in the 1960s, advocating that the changing culture toward physical attractiveness and beauty standards had negative health and psychological repercussions for fat individuals. Some believed that because the slim and fit body type had become the acceptable standard of attractiveness, those obese amongst us were going to great pains to lose weight and that this was, in fact, not always healthy for the individual.

Reporters then opined that **"slim, obese people"** experience physical and psychological harm as a result of dieting to levels below their ideal body weight.

Forced weight changes are not only likely to be short-lived, but they can also be harmful to the body and mind.

Emotional and destructive inclinations appear to be released during dieting whereas individuals were able to relax and feel better while maintaining their weight by eating normally.

The Kick Start ...

In the early 1980s, four books collectively put forward ideas related to **"Health at Every Size"** (HAES). In Diets Don't Work (1982), some believed this would result in weight loss as a side effect. Others further argued that everybody has a natural weight and set point; and that dieting for weight loss does not work.

The basic premise of HAES is that "well-being and healthy habits are more important than any number on the scale". Many experts promoted the idea of Health at Every Size for improving women's self-confidence and sexual well-being.

Social Media, a Boon or Bane?

While social media has many advantages, it also has some disadvantages, one of which is a rise in poor body image. In fact, several studies have discovered a link between how much time a person spends reading through social media, whether it's Facebook, Instagram, Snapchat, or Tik-tok, and how poorly they feel about their own body image. We hold unrealistic standards and feel even worse about ourselves.

How social media impacts mental health?

"89 percent of women reported feeling uncomfortable about themselves when they read comments on social media about other people's appearances".

A sample of 100 participants was drawn from different colleges and universities in the **Delhi/NCR** region of India. The probability-purposive sampling technique was used to select the two criteria groups, consisting of fifty males and fifty females. The data was analyzed with the help of descriptive and inferential statistics. It was found that females tend to use social media more for body comparison and report high concerns; however, they have lower self-esteem compared to their male counterparts.

The study may be used as a guide for our social media consumption treatments in the area of applied social psychology. The findings may offer a theoretical foundation for encouraging good body perception in the area of positive psychology. Social media is used for body comparison, self-esteem issues, and body image issues.

When you are constantly looking at imagery online that fits the ideals (models in advertisements, actors on TV, friends, or influencers with filtered photos), it can create the illusion that everyone barring you fits well into the narrow ideal.

To ensure that your worldview of body image is realistic, some researchers advocate expanding your social media exposure to include genuine, unfiltered human bodies of various shapes, sizes, and colours. They argue that doing so might help avoid harmful comparisons that create poor body image.

यत्र नार्यस्तु पूज्यन्ते रमन्ते तत्र देवताः ।

यत्रैतास्तु न पूज्यन्ते सर्वास्तत्राफलाः क्रियाः ।।

yatra nāryastu pūjyante ramante tatra devatāḥ

yatraitāstu na pūjyante sarvāstatrāphalāḥ kriyāḥ

"Where women are honoured, Divinity blossoms there;

where they are dishonoured, all actions remain untruthful."

-   Manusmriti 3/56

12. Drutanasan

(Addressing Fatphobia)

"Style Has No Size."

\- *Preetha Kkiran*

This is a form of bigotry that equates fatness with ugliness, inferiority and immorality.

Aside from social media, much of our exposure to negative body image beliefs comes from individuals around us – peers, family, friends, and co-workers. If a parent, grandparent, aunt, or uncle mentions how your body has recently changed, let her know right away that you don't like talking about appearance – or that your body is the least interesting thing about you – and you'd prefer to focus on discussing your hobbies, experiences, curiosities, and learnings. Or, if your friend expresses envy about another friend who has recently lost weight, remind them that all bodies are different and we don't know whether weight loss is a sign of something unhealthy.

These approaches show that by questioning these subtle but ubiquitous signals promoting body standards, we need to convey powerful messages to people around us that all bodies are excellent bodies.

13. Satahchittahanananda (I am fit)

SUTRA 3

1. Every day, tell yourself nice things, the efficacy of repeating to oneself encouraging statements helps improve one's body image. A great way to do this is to stand in front of the mirror each morning and compliment yourself on your looks or certain aspects of your body.

2. Take part in activities you avoid because of body image issues.

   Negative body image is a major barrier for a lot of people. A person could decide not to take certain photos on days when they feel overweight or unattractive, or they might decide not to go on a specific beach vacation out of anxiety that they won't look well in a bathing suit.

   NutritionOnUrPlate encourages our members to go all in and pursue what they desire, even when they believe their body image is holding them back.

3. Act as though you are confident in your body, and you will find that you are.

4. Move your body in fun ways. Exercise is good for our health in a variety of ways, and it may also help us develop a healthy body image.

5.   Take Your Attention Away from Weight

To battle poor body image, we suggest shifting attention away from weight, which may involve not weighing oneself frequently. Young individuals, particularly females, who constantly weigh themselves may suffer unfavourable emotional repercussions. All body sizes may be healthy, and everyone deserves delicious and nutritious cuisine regardless of size. Remember that body weight or size is not a behaviour while you attempt to develop the aforementioned health behaviours in yourself and/or your family.

6.   Dress for your current body type.

Body will change, whether or not something caused it to change, such as a life event like pregnancy.

Forcing oneself to "fit back into" clothes is not beneficial. *NutritionOnUrPlate* suggests treating your body with the respect it deserves by buying and wearing clothing that fits and complements it.

7.   Body acceptance is a more attainable objective for many people than body positivity. And it can prove extremely worthwhile in the long run too. Seek counselling from a health care provider if you continue to struggle with body image or your relationship with food. *NutritionOnUrPlate* is just a call away.

14. Indrajala

(The Magic Diet for Weight Loss)

The *Gita* calls for discipline and moderation in all spheres of life, as a means of healthy living. Consume the right kind of food to have inner and outer vitality, "*āyuh sattva*" - "that which promotes longevity".

Achieving the ideal healthy weight does not require a "diet" or "program", but rather a lifestyle that includes good eating habits, frequent physical exercise, and stress management. We have named it the "*No Diet*" diet plan for ease of understanding.

It's normal to desire to lose weight rapidly when you're attempting to do so. People who lose weight gradually and steadily are more likely to keep it off. Once you've reached a healthy weight, you can rely on proper food and physical exercise to help you stay healthy in the long run.

Losing weight is difficult and requires dedication. But if you're ready to get started, we've prepared a step-by-step guide to help you get started on the path to weight reduction and improved health. Before beginning the course, it is critical to approach the changes with compassion and to understand your preparedness and drive. You may attain your objectives by creating a supportive atmosphere, both physically and with the people in your life.

Even a little weight loss of 5% to 10% of your total body weight is likely to result in health advantages such as lower blood pressure, cholesterol, and blood sugar levels.

So, even if the ultimate goal appears daunting, consider it a journey rather than a destination. You will develop new food and physical activity habits that will assist you in leading a healthy lifestyle. These practices will assist you in maintaining your weight loss over time.

Losing weight requires dedication and a well-thought-out plan. Starting your weight reduction journey entails modifying your lifestyle to include a range of nutritious foods, frequent physical activity, adequate sleep, and stress management.

The billion-dollar weight control business and the widely held belief that being thin is more important than one's health are the main drivers of the epidemic of weight reduction regimens in our culture.

Weight loss and its management, the most trending topic on search engines, should be an extremely customized, disciplined, and maintainable routine. It should factor in the person's lifestyle, their health condition, disease burden, and most importantly – body capacity.

The challenge for Indians and perhaps with people all over the world is that their battle with weight steers them to trust every random source or influencer instead of relying on qualified dietitians.

15. Vikalpa Bhavanas

(Easy way not the Right one)

SUTRA 4

NutritionOnUrPlate is a proven platform that engages qualified nutritionists who are backed with the right educational credentials. They have the necessary experience similar to any other professional expert in their field - be it a doctor, an engineer or a chartered accountant that people reach out to. People who require our expertise will end up consuming random internet content but fail to evaluate if it can be applied to them verbatim.

During my many years in this profession, I have encountered numerous patients who have reported to my OPD complaining of extreme exhaustion and deficiency and it turns out that they had recently tried some method or diet to lose weight and crashed midway. Their bodies simply weren't up to it.

Many individuals across the world get obsessed with calorie counting, regulating macros, or avoiding specific meals to lose weight; nevertheless, these behaviours have several potentially harmful side effects.

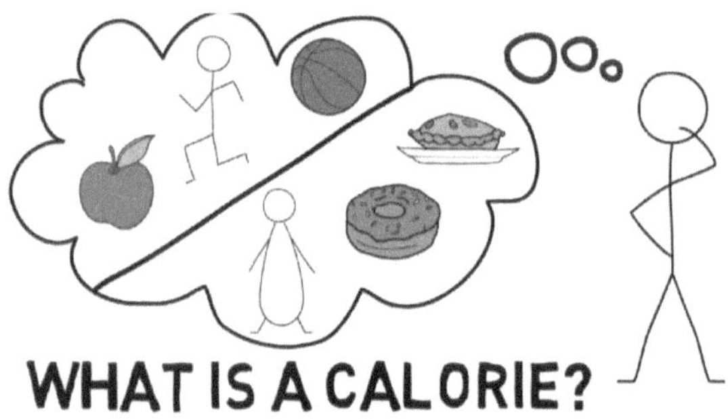

After the Covid 19 pandemic, it is quite alarming to see that post covid recovery, individuals are suffering from anorexia nervosa, an eating disorder characterised by abnormally low body weight, an intense fear of gaining weight and a distorted perception of weight. In many cases, we see individuals who rely on a single meal in a day, exercise for hours together and are in constant fear of putting on weight.

The Magic Diet is a healthy lifestyle that includes eating a good, balanced diet and engaging in physical activity that results in the desired side effect of weight loss. This is easier said than done. There are occasions when a person's obsession with losing weight may become all-consuming, turn into an overwhelming urge, and have severe effects on their daily life.

NutritionOnUrPlate cautions you that a lack of self-control when it comes to food, such as binge eating, burning more calories through exercise or cleansing, adhering to trendy diets like Yo-Yo diets, or weight swings. Some individuals develop an obsession with restricting their diet to foods that they believe to be high-quality or nutritious, whether that means they are organic, vegan, non-GMO, or something entirely different.

16. Pratipaksha Bhavana (Mindset)

"When it comes to eating, guilt has no place."

-   Preetha Kkiran

NutritionOnUrPlate has several research-backed programs that can aid in your recovery and from falling into the trap of dieting thus rebuilding your connection with food.

1. **Working with a qualified dietitian** or professional nutritionist is beneficial (preferably an IDA, CDE, IAPEN, or NSI member in India).

    We may assist you in breaking bad behaviours, substituting healthier objectives and concepts, and finally ditching the diet culture.

2. **Watch What You Eat**: your dietary habits should remain constant. No matter how your schedule changes, maintain a healthy eating regimen. For weekends, holidays, and special events, make plans in advance. Making a plan increases the likelihood that you'll have wholesome meals on hand in case your schedule changes.

3. **Breakfast every day is necessary**. Those who have lost weight and kept it off effectively share the practice of eating breakfast. By eating a healthy breakfast, you can avoid being "over-hungry" and overeating later in the day.

4. **Get some exercise each day**. People who have successfully lost weight and kept it off often engage in 60 to 90 minutes of moderate-intensity exercise without exceeding calorie demands. This does not

necessarily entail spending 60 to 90 minutes at once. It can include exercising for 20 to 30 minutes three times a day. For instance, taking a quick stroll in the morning, lunch, and evening. Before engaging in this degree of physical exercise, it may be useful to consult their doctor to ensure that any new changes are safe to proceed with.

Keep an eye on your nutrition and exercise. You can track your development and identify trends by keeping a log of your eating and physical activities. For instance, you could find that your weight gradually increases when you travel frequently for work or when you have to put in extra hours. When you become aware of this inclination, it might be a clue to try new things like bringing your own healthy food on the plane and scheduling time to work out while traveling. You might even do short laps around the building during your breaks.

5. **Be conscious of your weight**. Decide a weight check day of the week to track your progress. It's a good idea to monitor your weight when managing your weight reduction so that you may make the required adjustments to your food and exercise routine. If you've put on a few pounds, return to your original plan right away.

6. **Seek out the assistance of family**. People who have lost weight and kept it off successfully frequently rely on the encouragement of others to help them remain on track and get through any "bumps". This may even help you to stay motivated.

7. **Friends are forever**: if you have a buddy or partner who is also trying to lose weight or maintain their current weight reduction.

17. Svadhayaah

(One Adventure at a time)

"Do what makes you feel amazing."

- *Preetha Kkiran*

Making the decision to change your diet, lifestyle, and health is a big step. Start by personally committing to yourself. Writing down your motivations for wanting to lose weight will help you stay inspired. Regardless of whether you have a history of heart disease in your family, want to be an active participant in your child's wedding, or simply want to feel better in your clothing. Post these reasons where you'll see them every day, this will help you remember why you want to make this change. Keep a food record of everything you consume for a few days.

By doing so, you become more conscious of what you eat and when you consume it. This awareness might assist you in avoiding thoughtless eating. Tracking physical activity, sleep, and emotions; and keeping a food journal, will help you understand your existing habits and stressors. This will also indicate areas where you can make adjustments.

Next, consider your way of life. Identify potential obstacles to your weight loss attempts. Is it difficult to obtain adequate physical exercise because of your work or travel schedule? For example, do you find yourself eating sweet foods because you buy them for your children? Do your co-workers frequently bring high-calorie products to work, such as doughnuts, to share with everyone? Consider what you can do to assist in overcoming these obstacles.

If you are routinely reaching a certain goal, consider adding a new objective to help you stay on track. Reward yourself for your accomplishments! Recognize when you're on track and be happy with your accomplishments. Non-food incentives might be a bouquet of freshly selected flowers, a sports day with pals, or a soothing bath. Rewards might help you stay motivated in your quest to improve your health.

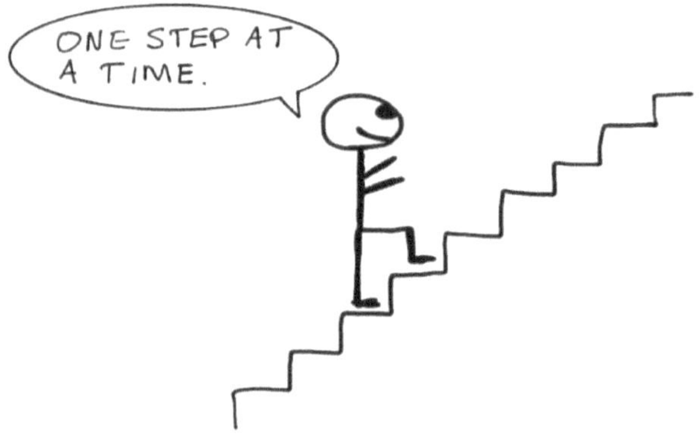

Many of us form habits when it comes to eating. Making abrupt, drastic adjustments, such as restricting yourself to a diet of cabbage soup alone might result in short-term weight reduction. However, such drastic adjustments are neither healthy nor wise, and they will fail in the long term. Permanently altering one's eating habits necessitates a methodical strategy that includes reflection, replacement, and reinforcement. Reflect on all of your distinct eating patterns, both healthy and unhealthy, as well as your typical triggers for unhealthy eating. Replace your bad eating habits with better ones. Renew your commitment to a better diet.

18. Praptabhuddhi (Be Smart)

सवादो पितो मधो पितो वयं तवा वव्रमहे ।

अस्माकमविता भव ।।

svādo pito madho pito vayaṃ tvā vavṛmahe

asmākamavitā bhava

"O pleasant Food, O Food of meath, thee have we chosen for our own,

So be our kind protector thou."

-   Rig Veda Mandala 1 Hymn 187

(translated by Ralph T.H. Griffith, 1896)

SMART stands for Specific, Measurable, Attainable, Realistic and Time-Bound

Choose a goal, identify your "why", make your goal smart, and measure your progress by how you feel.

The most important detail is that habit change can be achieved by selecting a long-term goal that will add positive aspects to your life.

To do this, it is important to identify a clear motivating force, or "why" to drive habit change.

This motivation will fuel you during times that feel challenging, and you may be more likely to achieve your end goal if there is a deeper connection to the end result.

The "why" should be fairly simple to answer, such as keeping up with your grandkids or feeling your strongest mentally and physically.

Internalize that motivation, and even consider writing it down. Continually connecting to your "why" is a great way to ensure that your motivation remains.

Small habits can add up to big changes over time, such as prepping up breakfast or lunch for the next day before you go to sleep.

Journaling for two minutes when you wake up or drinking a glass of water before a cup of coffee, active stretching for 5 minutes after each workout to improve flexibility and muscle recovery, incorporating speed work once per week, and daily recovery practices.

These steps include getting active, improving nutrition, losing weight, being mindful, and setting goals.

Getting active involves taking 10 minutes out of your day to take a walk, use an app to take a yoga class, or move in any way that feels right for you.

Improving nutrition involves adding one nutritious snack to your afternoon, and being mindful involves performing a five-minute guided meditation on an app while commuting. Setting goals is not always realistic, so don't be hard on yourself if you've made it halfway but feel like you want to go in a different direction.

The idea that food is only fuel and must be earned is a toxic notion that can lead to disordered eating and/or eating disorders. This is often seen after a major holiday when advertisements and articles push for detoxes or cleanses to "reset" or purge the body of "bad" food choices. However, not all physically beneficial components of food provide fuel.

Food is full of nutrients, phytochemicals, water, antioxidants, and other essential factors that contribute to an overall thriving body. Avoiding nutrient-dense foods in favour of low-calorie foods or restricting your food intake so that you do not obtain the correct amount of nutrients for optimal functioning can prove detrimental to your health in the long run and contribute to poor overall health.

Once you've adopted a few small, positive habits, you're likely to create lasting change.

Any meal or beverage whose recipe has been changed to minimize fat, carbs, and/or sugar to make it a component of a weight reduction program or diet is referred to as "**diet food**" (or "dietetic food").

Although bodybuilding supplements are made to make you gain weight, these meals are often meant to help you lose weight or modify the way your body looks. There is some debate about whether the sugar replacements used in diet meals that replace sugar with lower-food-energy alternatives might be hazardous. Artificial sweeteners have been under close study for decades, but the National Cancer Institute and other health organizations claim that there is no solid scientific evidence that any of the sweeteners that have been authorized for use in food or beverages cause cancer, but the jury is out on this one.

In many low-fat and fat-free foods, the fat is replaced with sugar, flour, or other full-food-energy ingredients, and the reduction in actual food energy value is small, if any.

19. Deepo Bakshayatey Dwanth

(Diet culture)

"When you strictly restrict how much food you can consume, it usually makes you want more of that meal in general."

- Preetha Kkiran

Diet culture is one factor that contributes to disordered eating habits, as it can lead to a lack of focus on nutrition while prioritizing low-calorie foods. This can have detrimental consequences, such as a greater risk of obesity and eating disorders, bone loss, gastrointestinal disturbances, electrolyte and fluid imbalances, low heart rate and blood pressure, increased anxiety and depression, and social isolation.

Mitahara, a concept in the Indian philosophy of Yoga, literally means the habit of moderate food. This integrates awareness about food, drink, balanced diet and consumption habits and its effect on one's body and mind.

There is no clinical definition for disordered eating, but it is most often described as a pattern of abnormal eating behaviours and thought patterns around food that do not yet fit the criteria for an eating disorder.

Diet culture is the belief that appearance and body shape are more important than physical, psychological, and even general well-being. It promotes thinness, aligns lower weights with higher moral virtues, and normalizes labelling foods and habits as good or bad.

This can lead to poor self-image, negative self-talk, and an all-or-nothing mentality, which can lead to disordered eating and depression. Diet culture is a social expectation that tells us how we should eat and look, and that if our bodies look a certain way – we are more accepted. This is dangerous and could harm people of all sizes, sex, and age. There are many different diets out there which are confusing, restrictive, and overwhelming.

Registered dietitians and nutritionists are essential to the detection and treatment of disordered eating, as many people are unaware that their eating patterns are problematic or harmful.

Unhealthy obsession can also lead to an eating disorder called orthorexia, which is an extreme form of clean eating that focuses on what the person believes to be the "correct" healthy diet.

Orthorexia is an eating disorder characterized by a restrictive diet, rituals based around eating, and the avoidance of foods not considered "good" or healthy. It can lead to other disorders such as anorexia nervosa and obsessive-compulsive disorders, as well as body dysmorphic disorder.

Diet culture contributes to orthorexia as it encourages avoiding foods or restricting your diet. Possible warning signs of orthorexia include compulsive checking of ingredient lists and nutrition facts labels, cutting out an increasing number of foods or food groups, showing high levels of distress when "healthy" foods aren't available, and obsessively following "healthy lifestyle" social media accounts and blogs. As with any pattern of disordered eating, orthorexia can interfere with an individual's mental and physical health and can lead to malnutrition when critical nutrients are eliminated from the diet.

It can also lead to an isolating disorder, as people with orthorexia feel virtuous when they eat foods, they consider good or safe, while deviating from their food restrictions causes anxiety and self-loathing. It is understood that this is a disorder known as orthorexia nervosa. Even if losing weight wasn't the main objective, it could happen as a result of orthorexia, a mental ailment that fits certain particular characteristics (eating disorder).

Anorexia, bulimia, and binge eating disorders are a few examples of eating disorders. Although it is not a diagnosis, the term "disordered eating" serves to describe aberrant eating behaviour.

Even if they don't fulfil the criteria for the current eating disorder diagnosis, someone might nonetheless have disordered eating habits. However, given its potential to develop into an even more severe eating disorder, disordered eating may still need to be treated. **Body dysmorphic** disorder causes people to become fixated and obsessed with their outward appearances and what they see as flaws.

Diet culture's belief systems view thinness as equal to health. These systems send the message that body types outside of a narrow range are considered unhealthy. News stories and social media often glamorize celebrity weight loss stories without questioning whether the methods used are healthy and sustainable.

Negative body image can be an effect of being teased, bullied, or criticized over your appearance or having a low or elevated body weight compared to others.

For some people, unrealistic goals can lead to an unhealthy body image and low self-esteem, as well as disordered eating behaviours. To have a healthy body image, you may require the help of a registered dietitian, nutritionist, psychologist, and/or other health care professionals.

The overall goal of any treatment is to help you accept your body and learn how to balance food and emotions. When used the right way, food is a source of pleasure, nourishment, and self-love. Read on to get a clear insight into the same. To overcome concerns about having a negative body image, a balanced eating pattern is necessary. The secret is to embrace a range of foods in moderation. Dietary limits were a result of diet culture.

Our presumption that our worth is determined by our physical appearance has given rise to a whole industry. The idea still holds true today. There is empirical evidence to support the claim that underweight individuals still diet because they are under pressure to lose weight. As already highlighted, people classify meals as "good" or "bad" based on whether they will (good) or won't (bad) satisfy the strict criteria set forth by diet culture.

Diet culture's harms are widespread. With diet culture in charge, we are expected to spend our valuable time, money, and energy in pursuit of looking a certain way and being "healthy" and "fit" enough. We are socialized to fail. We can earn our worth through weight and wellness. This distracts you from other important aspects of your life, such as work, education, relaxation tips, and rest.

Culture also contributes to the prevalence of eating disorders which have the highest mortality rates of any mental illness. It's estimated that up to 30 million people have an eating disorder in the United States alone. About 30% students have abnormal eating attitude, about 42.7% have suspected eating disorder. Well known eating disorder risk factors, such as body image dissatisfaction, weight stigma, and a history of dieting, are par for the course in diet culture.

While diet culture harms everyone, its effects are especially detrimental to marginalized groups. That's because diet culture reinforces existing systems of oppression.

Diet culture is harming us in more ways than one

It assumes thin and visibly "fit" as healthy and desirable. This ignores the reality of body diversity and perpetuates widespread fatphobia. Diet culture also has roots in classism. It pushes a mandatory "**wellness culture**" with prohibitive costs while ignoring issues like poverty and food availability. Further, diet culture is ableist in its insistence that we can all be "healthy" and stave off disease if we just buy the right foods, take the right supplements, and commit to the right exercise routine.

This is not an exhaustive list of the harm that diet culture causes or the types of oppression that it supports, but it does provide a foundation for helping you understand that when diet culture is the norm, we all lose.

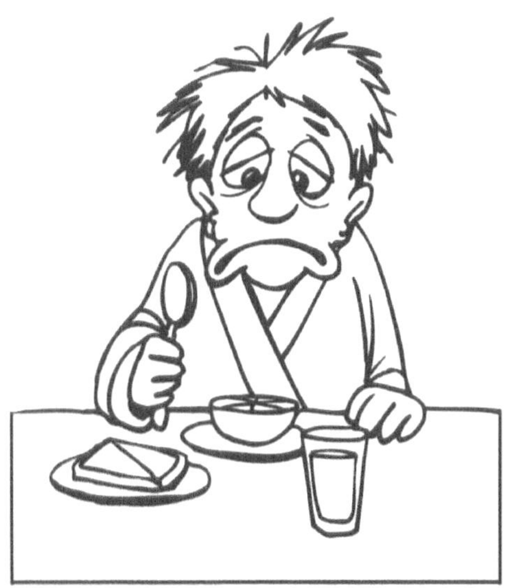

20. Annam Na Nindath

(Intuitive Eating)

"We can look within and return to a position of body trust through the skill of Intuitive Eating, which allows us to unlearn diet culture."

- *Preetha Kkiran*

A non-diet technique called "Intuitive Eating" which we call *the "No Diet" diet* at *NutritionOnUrPlate* can help you forget societal norms about what to eat and instead train you to pay attention to your own hunger cues.

This method of eating called Intuitive Eating, including how the body reacts to signals of hunger and contentment. With this method, concentrating on "weight control" is discouraged. Additionally, by taking a holistic approach to these topics and cancelling the toxic diet culture, Intuitive Eating tries to alter consumers' perceptions of what they know about dieting, health, and well-being. A good attitude and relationship with food, exercise, and the body are also fostered by the *"No Diet"* diet plan.

Our diet through Intuitive Eating believes that there is no such thing as "good" or "bad" food and does not attempt to restrict or eliminate certain meals. Instead, practitioners are urged to pay attention to their bodies and consume what feels healthy to them.

Let us get our focuses on concepts that include rejecting the diet mentality, embracing hunger, coming to terms with food, facing the food police, feeling full, discovering the joy element, honouring our body, controlling our emotions without resorting to food splurging, exercising, and taking care of our health.

Ditch the Diet; Dare to Define has outlined a few fundamental ideas to assist you in developing a better relationship with food and self-care.

By bringing to your attention - the false promises offered by the diet culture, Intuitive Eating can assist you in rejecting the diet mentality. It enables you to stop categorizing foods as "good" or "bad".

Learn to exercise for enjoyment rather than calorie restriction, and get rid of the "eating" guilt.

Read on if your eating behaviours are controlling your thoughts, interfering with your daily activities, or becoming overpowering.

A 2022 review done by *NutritionOnUrPlate* found that Intuitive Eating helped decrease dieting and concerns about weight. This review correlated with self-esteem and self-compassion, and lead to improved quality of life, body image, and body appreciation.

According to a 2019 Indian study which we referred, women who adopted Intuitive Eating habits were able to let go of the idea of "good" and "bad" meals, which are frequently encouraged by diet culture, and were able to maintain a diet that was more wholesome, sustainable, and non-restrictive.

Registered dietitians including yours truly will warn you that this "non-diet" approach will yield different results for different people who choose to follow this method of eating; no two bodies are the same, and no two people will react to the same diet.

It is important to point out that people with certain medical issues can have a specific diet given to them by their professional consultants, which would obviously preclude them from choosing an Intuitive Eating plan.

Counter claims about Intuitive Eating have been made that since the concept of Intuitive Eating is so broad and there is no fixed diet or food limitation. It might be challenging for certain people to know how much food to consume. Understanding one's hunger and fullness cues might take some time and practice. Please read on to get more clarity on the same.

21. Ashtanga Sunskruthi

(To Define You)

"When you give up diet culture, you finally have the space to understand more about yourself."

- *Preetha Kkiran*

SUTRA 5

8 propositions for implementing *"No Diet"* diet plan

Nutritional support for your health is a fantastic objective. For most of us, diet and food restriction guidelines can be perplexing, making the act of eating a meal a stressful experience. Trade your diet for sustainable nutrition habits to regain trust around food and retain the focus on health and well-being rather than cutting out foods or adopting restrictive practices.

Developing long-term eating habits is a more sustainable strategy than a fad diet and is typically healthier for your mental and physical health. Tips for breaking free from diets and creating sustainable nutrition habits that enhance your overall health are…

1. **Examine your current habits.**

   One of the least sustainable practices that individuals occasionally adopt unknowingly is radically overhauling what they're presently doing. Making abrupt, drastic changes can be inspiring, but they are more difficult to maintain. Making tiny alterations to your present routines, on the other hand, may be easier to adapt to and maintain.

   For example, if you already cook your lunch at home rather than going out to eat, supplement it by carrying snacks such as fresh fruit, yoghurt, almonds, or homemade *ladoos*. If you prefer cereal or *pohe / upma / idlies* for breakfast, consider mixing in some yoghurt and fruit or nuts for extra protein and minerals.

2.   Begin with a strategy.

A plan can help you build a structure for long-term eating habits. A strategy does not need to be overly comprehensive or stringent. Planning is a strategy that can help relieve the stress of making on-the-spot decisions.

Whether you want to follow an eating plan like the Mediterranean, DASH, or MIND diet or create your own using the ICMR NIN recommendations, having a rough notion of how you want to eat can help you make decisions.

It is important to note that these eating plans are neither all-inclusive nor restrictive but rather provide broad guidance on what sorts of foods promote specific health outcomes and goals, such as improving heart or brain health and maintaining a healthy weight.

3.   Make it long-lasting.

Whatever strategy that you devise, it should be one that you can see yourself following in the long run. This does not imply tight adherence or never eating things that are not generally consumed in your plan, but rather the capacity to keep eating in a way that promotes your health and objectives in the long run.

Creating practices that support your eating style can assist you in doing this. Meal planning and preparation, deciding on a number of meals that you would love to eat outdoors, and pre-planning sweets and delights to fit into a balanced eating plan are some examples. Meal planning has been linked to increased nutritional diversity and higher-quality eating habits, and it is a great way to boost the sustainability of your nutrition practices.

4.   Take note of your body's cues.

Your body is quite good at telling you when you're hungry. However, if you've recently dieted or if overeating has transformed into a habit, you may be out of touch with your hunger and fullness cues.

If you've been dieting for a long period of time, hormones like ghrelin will send signals that increase hunger and encourage you to seek food to escape starvation. Relearning or tuning into your body's cues might help you eat the right quantity of food.

The *"No Diet"* diet or Intuitive Eating refers to listening to your body's cues and using them to select what and when to eat. You may practice this by using a hunger and fullness scale, where you never allow yourself to be hungry below a 3 out of 10, and you stop eating when you reach a fullness level of 6. Then wait approximately 20 minutes to see if you want more food or if your body is telling you that it's had enough.

5. Food Restriction

It bears emphasizing that regardless of how you choose to eat, what plan you choose, or what habits you form, there is no requirement to adhere to any of them to the letter. In actuality, occasionally straying from the plan is a healthy and balanced way of living.

Every culture relies on food options that go well beyond just supporting life. Food is meant to be enjoyed. Food is both happy and comforting, and it fosters memories and a sense of community. It is essential to shift away from considering food as merely necessary for survival and towards seeing it as an enjoyable component of life.

6. Plan Your Eating Out Experience.

If you like dining out but are concerned about how it could fit into a healthy lifestyle, you can come up with some tactics for eating out while feeling good about your choices. Remember that the occasional decadent supper out is entirely okay and even excellent for long-term nutrition that benefits your emotional and physical well-being.

However, if you frequently dine out and want to avoid some of the meals and dishes that leave you feeling depleted of energy or nourishment, try to prepare ahead. Check the menu online ahead of time to decide on a meal or side dishes. You may include items you enjoy, such as a delicious burger or steak, and substitute steamed broccoli for fries, simple and good idea.

7. Make sure you have fun with it.

Long-term success requires that you enjoy your meals. If you don't appreciate what you eat, you're more inclined to give up and consume additional comfort foods. There's no reason to push yourself to consume foods you don't enjoy, no matter how nutritious they are.

If you want to eat more green vegetables but don't like kale or spinach, try various greens until you discover one you like or a nice way to prepare it, such as in a smoothie. However, if you can't find a version you like, skip it entirely. There is no one sort of food that you must consume to be healthy.

8. Include Exercise.

Exercise is an essential component of a healthy lifestyle. Exercise has several advantages that extend far beyond weight loss. Exercise boosts your chances of reaching and maintaining a healthy weight. Exercise also reduces appetite and might be a helpful method if you want to lose weight.

Make sure your long-term dietary patterns complement your activities, including getting in the right amount of calories to encourage energy production and tissue repair.

Extreme lifestyles and fad diets can be alluring, especially if the advertising makes bold assertions. Any food regimen that is too severe, too meticulous, or one you can't picture yourself maintaining over the long term will fail.

We, at *NutritionOnUrPlate*, have seen a third to two-thirds of dieters gain back more weight than they initially lost when following fad diets. Restrictive eating patterns can raise the risk of eating disorders, body dissatisfaction, osteoporosis, psychological stress, physical health problems, depression, and low self-esteem.

You will reap significantly more long-term benefits from a balanced, healthy diet. If you're having trouble creating a diet that works for you, think about speaking with a licensed dietician.

22. Navyasiddhant

(Is this the ordinance?)

"I won't compromise my mental well-being in order to acquire the ideal physique."

-   *Preetha Kkiran*

What are the food regulations? What rules apply to food? And how to break them

These standards are frequently strict and might have an impact on how we feel about ourselves. When we identify food as excellent or awful, we also label the act of eating it. We then begin to internalize our own values as a result of our eating habits. This can result in a tangled connection between food and our bodies.

Food regulations are more widespread than you would imagine. Even minor restrictions, such as "no eating after 8 p.m." might be called food rules. While not all of them are immediately damaging, being conscious of the eating rules you follow is beneficial. Numerous elements have an impact on food restrictions. Your family, culture, the cuisine you can eat, and the lessons society has taught you are all important considerations that result in you placing stringent limitations on what you can eat.

Family Opinions and Upbringing is key. What was modelled for you as a child has a huge influence on how you view eating. If you have a parent or family member who has a bad connection with eating, you are likely to have the same perspective. A parent's eating habits are passed on to their offspring. These practices include pressure to finish your entire portion, belief driven restrictions and such. All of these practices have the potential to result in the development of food regulations.

Food Rules Examples: Most Indian families follow certain customs, which their children typically continue as they mature into adults. Food is no different, nor are eating practices. You could be tempted to do the same if your family ate (or didn't eat) a certain way.

Here is a list of certain dietary rules that may be passed down through families: Food should be taken off the plate. Each day, you must eat three square meals. Only eat when you are truly hungry, Toss out the carbs, munch just bittersweet chocolate. Food laws may differ greatly in terms of what is actually good for your health and what isn't.

The most important thing is to comprehend the purpose of your dietary restrictions and how they meet your current needs for nutrition and mental wellness.

23. Mansmritih

(Mindful eating/Awareness)

"When you eat mindfully, you slow down, pay attention to the food you're eating, and savour every bite."

- *Preetha Kkiran*

In the wellness market, it's sad but safe to say that there will always be a new fad diet. It's also reasonable to conclude that, while promising to address all of your health problems with a single fast and easy purchase or hack, these diets are unlikely to be a long-term answer to your health goals. Dieters recover more than half of the weight they lost within two years. But it's not simply weight fluctuations that might arise from fad diets, other lifestyle factors and behaviours can also have a long-term influence.

While there are certainly expert-approved eating regimens that may assist people in reaching (and maintaining) their weight and health objectives in a safe and sustainable manner, the National Institute of Health indicates that dieters are five times more likely to develop an eating problem.

What about people on calorie-restricted diet? Their chances of having an eating disorder skyrocket.

Diet culture, in reference to the most recent fad diet or weight-loss product, has an agenda, creating "issues" with our bodies that can subsequently be rectified, studies indicate that more than 95% of diets are unsuccessful. When our diet fails, it directly affects our self-esteem since dieting can be so time-consuming, with all of the planning, calorie monitoring, and self-control necessary.

In addition to having negative impacts, shame over dietary "failure" can cause harmful behaviours like limiting, purging, or over-exercising in an effort to alleviate the guilt. These are abnormal behaviours that have the potential to develop into very serious eating disorders.

24. Swatmanambhoddah (Consciousness)

"There's enough on this planet for everyone's needs but not for everyone's greed."

— *Mahatma Gandhi*

Very good food is generally more expensive and not as readily accessible in all locales. These "good" foods can be significantly out of reach in food deserts, which are typically concentrated in black and brown neighbourhoods. Consider the food that has been labelled as "bad" or "to be avoided". These meals are often cheaper and widely available in all locations. Furthermore, meals associated with people of colour have historically been seen as "bad" or "unhealthy" by the west.

Many food rules are designed with a more affluent, mostly white, populace in mind. This is so because "healthy" cuisine is typically associated with white, western cultures; for example, grilled chicken, brown rice, and vegetables are often listed as the average diet meal. How can you circumvent food laws? Creating a healthy relationship with food is a prerequisite for breaking eating norms. Think about how these regulations affect your life. Do they make you feel bad? Do they prevent you from enjoying life? How would it feel to break these laws? Engage in an introspective practice while avoiding judgment. The ***"No Diet"*** diet is also an excellent way to break free from food rules. Our bodies are designed to communicate with us about what we need. When we get caught up in eating restrictions, we might lose touch with our bodies and their signs. Try to be aware of your hunger cues and when they appear, pay heed to them.

Intuitive Eating is a healthy approach to controlling weight and a valuable skill for preventing disordered eating; seek professional assistance if your eating rules become burdensome. There are professionals who can guide and support you as you embark on a new relationship with food and your body; any restrictive eating guidelines might have a detrimental impact on you.

To break those norms, you must study the meals you love and figure out how to improve your connection with them. Intuitive Eating (*"No Diet"* diet approach) professional coaching are ideal starting points for developing a positive body image and a balanced relationship with food. If you continue to have a bad attitude towards food and your connection with it, consult an expert. That is why, in response to the culture of dietary limitation and constraint, many nutrition and psychology professionals are exploring the concept of "food freedom".

25. Pralobahnad Vimuktih

(Break Free!)

"To re-establish healthy control, Get rid of harmful control."

- *Preetha Kkiran*

NutritionOnUrPlate, which specializes in eating disorders and chronic dieting says - Independence from food is not a diet. It is the mindset of nourishing your body organically without feeling like your decisions are impacted by the "should" that we commonly internalize from diet culture. An illustration of this would be letting yourself eat a piece of double cheese pizza (or two, depending on how hungry you are) for lunch today since you aren't evaluating your value in relation to what or how much you consumed.

When you are in a state of **food independence**, you don't second-guess your choices and understand that you can rely on your body to guide you. Dietary independence does not imply a disrespect for healthful foods; it simply allows for more flexibility, variety, and indulgence while honouring hunger, fullness, and cravings and letting go of foods that were previously considered off limits. Food independence provides an alternative to dieting and all of its associated baggage.

Ultimately, eating flexibility gives us more freedom in other areas of our lives. Having a food freedom attitude implies you can't fail. When food isn't on your mind, eating something unusual doesn't have the same power to make you feel so guilty, freedom to eat what you want, when you want, means you can never slip up. Restrictive dieting can cause the metabolism to slow down.

In fact, research published in the journal Obesity followed up on **The Biggest Loser Competitors** six years after intense crash diets and discovered that their damaged metabolisms never entirely recovered. While food independence is not explicitly a weight loss technique, it does not exclude the two from coexisting. There is some emerging evidence suggesting that Intuitive Eating is beneficial for weight maintenance.

According to research published in the journal Eating Disorders, there is a clear link between Intuitive Eating and self-reported weight stability, as well as overall body acceptance and a lesser desire for weight change. Those who had a food freedom perspective were less likely to have disordered eating habits, body dissatisfaction, depressive symptoms, and low self-esteem.

If you're worried about not being able to do it "right", know that food freedom is different for everyone because we all have different food experiences. Take heart in the fact that we don't have to love our weight, shape, or appearance in order to find food freedom. A smart starting step is to assess your present restrictions and examine where they came from. There could be food rules that you are breaking without even realizing it. Are there any specific foods, or even entire aisles, that you avoid when you go grocery shopping? Allow yourself to experiment with adding more diversity to your diet, and remember that it's alright to start small.

All sorts of food have a role in our lives. Of course, including nutrient-dense foods in our diet is important, but so is being able to enjoy a birthday cake with friends and family. Giving oneself unconditional permission to eat while re-learning your body's hunger, fullness, and wanting cues, which can be repressed with long-term dieting, is the first step in allowing this mentality to take root. Dieting requires a lot of mental work.

When you allow your brain to think about things other than food and weight, you expand the measures you use to evaluate your self-worth. Practice listing good traits about yourself that aren't related to weight or appearance – and, to take it a step further, clean up your social media.

Unfollow an account if you feel it makes you feel bad about your body or food, surround yourself with people who share your values, Food should be enjoyed! Many studies have demonstrated that social support helps people achieve their physical activity and exercise objectives, and the same is true for food modification.

A 2021 research published in Public Health Nutrition found that having a supportive social network helps people achieve their healthy eating objectives. We live in a world that values diet culture and the slender ideal, making it difficult to be satisfied with our looks. This can leave us feeling like we've failed or that if we just tried harder, our bodies and self-image would improve. It might also be challenging to break free from this cultural perspective. Food independence is a long-term goal, and it's appropriate to do it slowly and with encouragement.

If you're having trouble, *NutritionOnUrPlate* recommends reaching out to a therapist or registered dietician specializing in Intuitive Eating and disordered eating recovery to support you in your journey.

26. Atangika Margah

(Eightfold path)

SUTRA 6

Weight loss is a popular objective in the wellness industry. However, focusing too much on the scale might be harmful to your mental health, causing you to overlook important parts of overall wellness. Instead of focusing on a number, shift your emphasis to setting objectives for wellness and behaviour modification.

Wellness objectives should centre on improving your mind, body, and soul. Small behavioural adjustments might result in significant advantages. After all, achieving good and long-term health requires a variety of health-promoting behaviours.

Making modifications is not straightforward. You've been living a particular way for a long time, and your go-to tools are presumably ones you picked up along the way. They may have worked in the past, but sometimes changes are required for positive progress. Now that you've decided to set wellness objectives, it's time to figure out what you want to concentrate on. Because it takes an average of 66 days to create a new habit, you'll want to give yourself plenty of time and resources to help you succeed. Use the **SMART** criteria to help you define your goals: specific, measurable, attainable, realistic, and timely.

Instead of saying, "I'm going to sleep more", try saying, "I'm going to bed 30 minutes earlier for 5 days a week over the next 4 weeks". The more specific your goals are, the more likely you are to achieve them. It is not necessary to move more through organized exercise.

Non-exercise activity includes any activity or movement that does not involve sport or exercise. Doing more physical tasks for yourself is not only healthy for the mind, but it also contributes significantly to your physical health. This is referred to as **NEAT** or Non-Exercise Activity Thermogenesis. NEAT can not only assist you in maintaining a good level of physical fitness but basic actions such as cleaning and decluttering can also enhance your quality of life and reduce stress. On-Exercise Activity Objectives include

* Instead of taking the lift to work, take the stairs.

* Hand-wash your car once a week.

* Instead of emailing a co-worker, walk over to their workstation.

* Stand up more. Consider using a standing desk. Simply standing during things that you would typically perform while sitting.

* For transit, walk or ride a bike.

* Have fun with your children.

* Do some garden work or cleaning around the house.

* Do an active family excursion once a week or as frequently such as hiking, bicycling, kayaking, paddle boarding, or making an obstacle course.

27. Nindra Saihithah (Sleep)

नक्तंचर्या दिवास्वप्रं आलस्यं पैशुनं मदम् ।

अतियोगमयोगं च श्रेयसोऽर्थो परित्यजेत् ॥

naktaṁcaryā divāsvapnaṁ ālasyaṁ paiśunaṁ madam atiyogamayogaṁ

ca śreyaso'rtho parityajet

"Persons who are willing for good health should not indulge in keeping awake at nights, sleeping in daytime, laziness, addiction of bad things and other such factors"

Nobody enjoys being sleep-deprived. **Sleep deprivation** not only makes you feel foggy and weary during the day, but it is also a key contributor to stress, decreased quality of life, mental discomfort, pain, weight gain, mood disorders, and other chronic health problems.

Making the decision to improve your sleep hygiene is not an easy task. Let's face it, there are occasions when you can't sleep because of circumstances beyond your control. Prioritizing sleep is well worth the effort if you believe it is achievable or if you have some wiggle room.

Gaining more sleep has several benefits, like hormone regulation, metabolic management, enhanced mental clarity and mood, optimal immune system function. Prioritize sleep, first decide what you want to accomplish, then figure out how to get there. "I will, five days a week, go to bed 30 minutes early and switch off screens one hour before bed". The next step is to put your strategy into action.

Set aside time for media breaks. Don't you simply love it when your phone or tablet informs you how many hours and minutes you've spent on your phone or tablet today? Devices may be all-consuming, and our screen time often reflects this.

While social networking has certain advantages, it may also generate a lot of tension and anxiety. Taking a pause to relax and reset the mind is not only a good idea but it has also been found to boost well-being and aid with sleep.

It does not have to be a lengthy time away from social media to be beneficial. Even a one-week break can result in considerable gains in well-being, despair, and anxiety. Develop a Creative Outlet with so many tasks to complete in a single day, it's easy to see why finding time for hobbies feels unattainable. So, if you can't find the time, make it yourself. We, at *NutritionOnUrPlate*, believe engaging in hobbies that you like, such as painting, dancing, and crafting, might help you live longer.

Developing a creative outlet is also beneficial to your mental health, particularly in a social context.

People who engaged in leisure activities had higher mental health than those who solely engaged in social activities. When the two were combined – leisure activities in a group setting or with a friend – mental health increased as well. Whether you have someone to craft with or not, making time for nurturing a creative outlet is a powerful tool for nourishing your well-being.

Everyone has gone through a period in their lives when they felt like they were just going through the motions. During everyday duties, it's easy to get overwhelmed and zone out. Being intentional and thoughtful throughout the day has a way of calming you down and bringing you down to earth. Our experience through years have revealed that the impacts of mindfulness go beyond having intention, but can help your psychological wellbeing as well.

Focusing on what you're doing is one way to stay present. Take note of how your arms move and how you breathe, straighten your upper body, push your shoulders back, or sit comfortably. Concentrate on relaxing and releasing stress. Keep an open mind and be patient. It is your responsibility to bear testimony to your own acts and experiences. Finding significance in life may have a significant impact on your health. Whether you are passionate about a particular cause or love volunteering to help others, experts have shown that doing so is an excellent technique for enhancing health and quality of life.

Making new acquaintances is difficult. There is no doubt about that. Making friends as an adult might be even more difficult. Fostering social relationships is more than simply finding someone to hang out with – it helps your entire health! Spending time with individuals you like might boost your mood and overall health.

Short-term and long-term social contacts have been proven in studies to lower the risk of cardiovascular disease, cancer, poor immunological function, and depressive symptoms; the impacts of loneliness and social isolation might be harmful. We have even linked it to obesity, smoking, alcohol consumption, and a lack of exercise.

Making an attempt to socialize with family, friends, and others on a daily or weekly basis at least once a week is a good place to start and maybe more achievable for those with hectic schedules.

Getting outside more often offers healing aspects as well as mental health advantages. Living and working near green areas has been linked to decrease in stress, sadness, and anxiety levels. Even if you live in the city, spending time outside will help you too.

28. Siddhi Praptah (Goal)

अमृतत्वस्य तु नाशास्ति वित्तेन ।

amṛtatvasya tu nāśāsti vittena

"Immortality cannot be achieved by wealth"

> \-   *Sage Yajnavalkya to Sage Maitreyi*
> *Brihadaranyaka Upanishad*

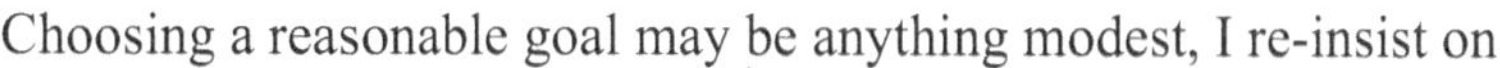

Choosing a reasonable goal may be anything modest, I re-insist on

- Spending 10 minutes outside during your lunch break, five days a week.

- Going for a stroll after dinner, three evenings a week are also good ways to start.

- Take a walk or ride your bike three times per week.

- Read a book while sitting beneath a tree at least once in 3 months.

- Consider stargazing or cloud viewing once a week.

- Park a little further away from your destination every day.

It is a marathon, not a sprint, to work on improving your health.

While getting on the scale is perhaps the most popular method of measuring success, it is not necessarily the greatest.

Non-weight-loss wellness goals can have a significant impact on your health and well-being.

Change does not occur overnight. Speaking with a healthcare practitioner, counsellor, or registered dietitian can assist you in developing realistic objectives that are appropriate for you and your lifestyle.

29. Navarambh

(The Next Big Thing)

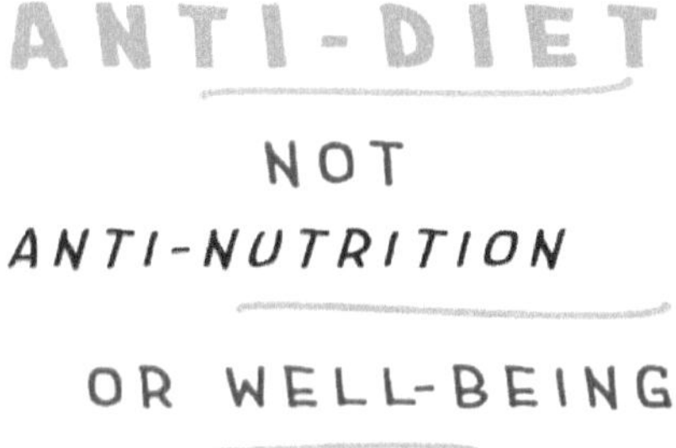

The philosophy of "health at every size" and the anti-diet movement are closely related. Creating a mentally healthy relationship with food, promoting body acceptance, and eradicating fatphobia and stigma from our culture are the goals of this strategy and movement. India has become quite stigmatized as a result of the **"War on Obesity"**. For a variety of reasons, people fear being overweight. Many individuals are instructed to avoid being overweight at all costs, whether it's due to societal stigma or worry about their health.

This has resulted in dieting, anxiety about eating, a negative connection with food, using exercise as a form of discipline, purging, starvation, and other behaviours. These factors can all result in unneeded emotional, mental, and bodily suffering. Furthermore, it has been shown that many of the weight-loss techniques used today fail. It has been observed that dieting might lead to an obsession with eating. This causes people to categorize foods as "good" or "bad" and to view eating as a system of rewards and punishments. This kind of thinking frequently produces emotional, mental, and bodily suffering, sometimes even resulting in disordered eating patterns.

Intuitive Eating is a goal of the anti-diet movement. Intuitive Eating places a strong emphasis on only eating when you are hungry and only eating until you are satisfied. This entails assessing environmental elements, signals, and feelings. Furthermore, the emphasis is shifting away from body weight and food labels and towards overall wellbeing.

Validating your present moment experience while also being able to analyze it can help people recognize whether they are truly hungry or full or if external factors are causing them to reject or want food. Sadly, this is the challenge that every other individual is facing today and needs in-depth analysis to move forward.

I want you to question yourself - "Am I really on Continual dieting?", if you have unusual eating habits, chronic weight changes, food/weight/body image obsessions, food-related feelings of shame, remorse, or loss of control, punishment via exercise, dietary restriction, fasting, or purging?

The Anti-Diet movement's recommended technique, Intuitive Eating, has been found to enhance behavioural and psychological health in a number of contexts. Additionally, it is regarded as an effective strategy for enhancing mental health and lowering problematic eating patterns. Combating unhealthy eating behaviours and promoting greater mental and emotional health are its key goals.

Contrary to popular belief. *NutritionOnUrPlate*'s anti-diet practices take into account both exercise and nutrition, as is the case with many wellness programs. In actuality, the anti-diet movement encourages engaging in physical activity for enjoyment, which has a number of advantages.

Your cardiovascular health, workout retention, body image, and connection with food may all be enhanced by engaging in regular exercise. According to several studies, anti-diet behaviours might enhance cardiometabolic risk and quality of life even in the absence of weight reduction. A healthy relationship between food and body image is just as crucial as a healthy relationship with exercise. Poor eating and body image habits have a disproportionately negative influence on women, who are the subject of several studies.

For women who struggle with weight and body image, anti-diet practices have been demonstrated to improve eating, weight, and psychological variables. However, women are not the only group that is negatively impacted by weight and body image. Children are another demographic that is severely impacted by weight prejudice. In addition to being mentally impacted, children who suffer from weight bias are likely to participate in dangerous weight-related behaviours. Anti-diet behaviours can help kids and teenagers avoid disordered eating and enhance their general health as they get older.

30. Punnaravrittih (Ditch the Diet)

Don't dig your grave with your own knife and fork.

-   *Old English Proverb*

If you wish to start living an anti-diet lifestyle, and follow the *"**No Diet**"* diet, start by putting these strategies into practice:

When you're hungry, eat a meal, but be mindful of any emotions that might be affecting your hunger or lack thereof.

Put an end to "good" and "bad" food labelling.

Stop punishing yourself for your eating habits by restricting your diet and exercising more.

To stay in shape for fun, experiment with various forms of exercise like swimming, riding, or dancing.

Develop an appreciation for and care for yourself.

Acknowledge the requirements of your body.

Never start a diet unless medically necessary and is being overseen by a healthcare professional or a nutritionist.

Be mindful of the media you consume because much of it doesn't represent reality.

Be mindful of how you and others speak about your weight and body image.

It might be difficult to try to develop (or renew) a healthy connection with food and your body.

Be nice to yourself and understand that it may take some time to completely alter your viewpoint, actions, and ideas.

If you're striving to recover from an eating disorder, disordered eating, or a history of Yo-Yo dieting, the support of *NutritionOnUrPlate* can be a fantastic tool to help your recovery path.

However, you may start doing what is environmentally sound which I firmly believe in wherein I give suggestions for minimizing the effects of diets on the environment by limiting daily meat consumption to 70g per person, putting plant proteins first, encouraging the consumption of sustainable seafood, moderate dairy intake amongst others.

Putting a focus on starchy, whole-grain meals, promoting locally grown produce that is in season.

Reducing excessive eating of meals heavy in fat, sugar, and salt, encouraging the use of tap water and unsweetened tea or coffee as the default options for hydration.

Minimizing food waste.

31. Svastyah

(Best shape of one's life)

"Your goals, minus your doubts, equal your reality."

-   Ralph Marston

You're ready to **Ditch the Diet**…

- if you've spent the most of your life on diets and struggle to break the diet mentality.

- if you worry that as you get older, your connection with food and your body may deteriorate.

- if you want to regain your former body confidence.

- if you are prepared to make changes in your life and devote more time to your children so that dieting won't occupy as much of your valuable mental resources.

- if you're feeling lost and unsure of your next steps, but you know you need to break your diet-related habits.

- if **Now**! you are prepared to change your habits, even if it will be difficult, and you'll need an accountability partner who will refuse to let you fail.

- if you want to exercise because it's fun, not because you have to burn calories to stay on track.

With *NutritionOnUrPlate*'s customized program, you'll get the support, accountability, and expert coaching you need - to eat and exercise in a sustainable way without restrictive diets or spending your life in the gym endlessly.

What *NutritionOnUrPlate*'s *"No Diet"* diets could look like:

➢ Focus on choice, not calories.

➢ A meal plan with *"No Diet"* diets is never based on calories but instead focuses on variety and choice.

Making a decision about whether or not to eat something because of its caloric or nutrient content is a dieting behaviour. That mindset leads to restriction or avoidance of certain foods, while ignoring aspects of eating like pleasure and enjoyment. However, building in a variety in your grocery cart or planned recipes ensures you can still create balanced and nourishing meals.

➢ Include in abundance.

Fruits (fresh, frozen, canned, dried and 100% juice), Vegetables (fresh, frozen, canned, dried and 100% juice), Proteins (plant based or otherwise), Dairy, Grains or breads or starches, Beverages, and Snacks.

You alongside *NutritionOnUrPlate* can also think in terms of categories for organizing your kitchen and setting up an environment that supports efficiency. We can brainstorm options for your refrigerator, freezer, and pantry so you have a variety of shelf-stable options that can be used later as well as a choice of perishable, fresh items that should be used sooner. Meal planning and prepping also helps reduce food waste when you have a variety of items stocked and ready for when you need them!

➢ Minimize stress and chaos.

The *"No Diet"* diet plan can identify opportunities to shop and cook that fit into a chaotic schedule, eliminating stress or lastminute dashes to the grocery store. There's nothing more bothersome to me than browsing or driving back and forth across town looking for a specific ingredient or specialty item. That adds stress to my day, wastes my time, and leaves me feeling frustrated that I couldn't make do with what I had at home or find a simpler solution. That's part of why, in a very busy working lifestyle, I include a plan for when and where I shop so I can make just one trip to stock up on anything and everything I need. I know exactly how long it takes me to get there and back, and I can factor that into the total time commitment I need to prep things for the week.

➢ Leftovers are an option for convenience, but are designed to be refreshed in taste appealing ways.

Growing up, I tolerated them, but they were never the most exciting thing. Now, I actually look forward to the routine and comfort of leftovers. That may sound weird, but it's really not—if that's one night that I don't have to cook, that's less mess to clean afterwards. And avoiding boredom is easier when I make sure there's always a tasty way to turn leftovers into something I actually want to eat.

The convenience factor is there too, which is one of the most appealing parts of meal prepping or planning in the first place. Give yourself the chance to explore what would make leftovers appealing to you and don't be afraid to experiment! It's OK to stumble or feel unsure about whether you're doing everything "right". The fact is that there's no such thing as a perfect diet or perfect meal, so *"No Diet"* diet supports the process of continuously learning and adapting to what you need.

Just get there and cook some food! After all, "Happiness is Homemade" isn't it?

And if you know someone with questions about *"No Diet"* diet, be sure to recommend this book so they can **Ditch the Diet; Dare to Define** themselves.

Whether you want to Improve your health and fitness, Improve your fortitude, Build muscle, Trim body fat, Get energetic, have a happy and healthy pregnancy or even Return to exercise after giving birth safely; above all if you want to Improve your connection with food, whether you want to boost your self-confidence or do anything else, *NutritionOnUrPlate* with me, Preetha, will assist you throughout our 3-

month program. You'll receive a simple, step-by-step plan for developing nutrition, fitness, and mindset habits that will lead the way to reach your goal.

Rediscover the pleasures of eating to make peace with food. If you eat and exercise in a way that complements rather than controls your life, you can achieve life-altering results.

32. NutritionOnUrPlate

I, Preetha Kkiran at *NutritionOnUrPlate* and our team of doctors, physiotherapists, and psychologists are available five days a week to answer questions and help you navigate situations like eating while you're on vacation, making exercise substitutions so you don't aggravate your knee pain, or planning a workout with limited equipment options, getting ready for a milestone like getting engaged, graduation, starting an enterprise, getting married or any other leap in life; we will find the best path toward long-term results together in a way that works.

Learning to improve your nutrition without giving up the foods you love, exercise safely and effectively so you're getting maximum results from your workouts without burning yourself out, increase your confidence, love the way your body looks, feels, and performs and enjoy your life more than you ever thought possible, and you'll become the happiest, fittest, and strongest version of yourself, one step at a time.

Looking for your next diet program. In case it wasn't clear, we're ditching diets here. Say *"No Diet"* diet and Move Forward.

"If we could give every individual the right amount of nourishment and exercise, not too little or too much, we would have the safest way to health."

- *Hippocrates*

Together, once and for all, let's break the cycle of dieting that grips us as individuals and as a society, join hands with the *"No Diet"* diet now.

Ditch the Diet begins with a journey through the **Evolution of a Dieter**, looking closely at where body dissatisfaction and dieting begins and then explaining the way our body, mind, and spirit reacts keeping us trapped in a dieting - triggered eating - shame cycle.

I have taken a close look at the foundation of how to eat, which is necessary to build a positive and healthy relationship with food. This includes principles of intuitive and mindful eating, allowing yourself to eat, and body acceptance. We can then delve into the more concrete concepts of building lasting habits and what authentic nutrition truly involves.

By realigning our thought processes as they relate to food, nutrition, dieting, and health while learning how to listen to and trust our bodies, we can achieve peace with food and authentic health in our lives.

33. Summary

Ditch the Diet >>> Dare to Define >>> Desire to Do

Now that you have read the book, I am sure a lot of worry with regards to how you need to channelise your well-being is clear. However, to ease out minute confusions that may linger in your mind about the dietary approach for a wholesome life, here is a short summary of the right steps to implement.

SUTRA 7

Get Up Early 4:30 A.M. – 5 A.M. Every Day

We humans have an internal clock that maintains a cycle of events at a 24-hour interval. It is found that the body temperature is minimum at 5:00 AM, the sleep-inducing hormone Melatonin peaks at around 11:00 PM and starts declining as the night progresses. The hormone Cortisol that helps to withstand stress and traumas in life is secreted more during our sleep.

Exercise 1.5 – 2 Hours Per Week

People who are physically active exhibited a 30 – 40% reduction in relative risk of colon cancer and 20 – 30% women showed reduction in the relative risk of breast cancer.

Eat Till You Are Just Full – Avoid Overeating - 80% Principle

When you overeat, stomach expands to contain the food and hence puts pressure on other organs making you feel fullness, distended abdomen, sluggish or tired. The stomach produces hydrochloric acid to breakdown food, which is thrown back to food pipe causing heartburn, our body tries to metabolise extra calories leading to feeling temporarily hot or even dizzy.

Eat Mindfully – Kickstart Mind – Approach Positively

What we think while eating, positive or negative, how thankful we are for the food we eat, impacts on our psychology and also affects our digestion. The first phase or step of digestion, the cephalic phase (begins when we see, smell and think about food) only works when we are relaxed and paying attention to what we eat. On the other hand, stress shuts down digestion.

Fasting Once a Week – Empty Stomach – Full Heart

Overweight humans show that calorie restriction or fasting improves health outcomes including several cardiac risk factors (which might cause heart diseases), improving insulin (factor responsible for glucose metabolism) sensitivity and reduces oxidative damage to both DNA and RNA thus helping in healthy aging.

Stay Hydrated – Pure Water Runs Life

Water is the nature's best form of nectar for a disease-free body, mind and soul.

34. Eat, Eat, Eat

SUTRA 8

EAT food as close to its natural state as possible.

EAT foods for what qualities, nature, and nutrients they possess.

EAT real, whole, unrefined foods for what they have: a rich array of nutrients that promote health.

EAT only Whole grains (enriched and fortified flours and pastas with whole source).

EAT real fruits in lieu of dried fruit or fruit juice. Real fruit has vitamins, minerals, beneficial phenolic compounds, essential fatty acids, and many other valuable substances not found in refined fruit products.

EAT fresh vegetables as they have more vitamins and minerals rather than those that are canned or frozen if you have a choice.

EAT Virgin oils in opaque containers, such as virgin flaxseed, canola, and olive oil.

EAT cold-pressed Kachhi Ghani or Coconut oil as nutrients are preserved; refined supermarket vegetable oils and hydrogenated oils may contain harmful radicals.

EAT freshly prepared meats, better than ground, smoked or aged meats. Aged meat or meat that has been ground days ahead of time often has disease-causing oxidized cholesterol that is rarely found in fresh meat. If you want to consume ground meats buy the lowest-fat cut of meat you can and have it ground right before using. Completely avoid all aged meats, including aged steaks and sausages.

EAT fresh Seafood which is better than that which has been canned or smoked. The fresher the fish, the more intact its valuable fatty acids will be.

EAT raw or dry roasted nuts and seeds, oil-roasted nuts and seeds have added salt which can diminish health and cause degenerative disease.

EAT herbs and spices instead of artificial colourings and flavourings.

EAT raw, certified milk as it is better than homogenized, pasteurized milk if you have the facilities that provide it at your doorstep.

EAT ghee and butter better than margarine.

EAT fresh eggs that are rich in beneficial nutrients and are far better than chemical-laden egg substitutes.

EAT (drink) unfermented green tea that is richer in beneficial compounds than tea that has been processed into regular black tea.

EAT local foods that are home-cooked to relish our tradition and revive our culture.

35. Shloka Nishkarsh Samarpanam (Conclusion)

My book **Ditch the Diet; Dare to Define** wraps up here with the hope that each reader achieves the sole purpose of their life:

धर्मार्थकाममोक्षाणामारोग्यं मूलमुत्तमम्।

dharma-artha-kāma-mokṣāṇāṃ

ārogyaṃ mūlaṃ uttamaṃ

"Health is the core for acquiring the four objectives of living. Dharma-Duties/ actions that give us support, Artha- Material Wealth/possessions, Kama- Our Wishes/Desires, Moksha- Enlightenment/Free from all Attachments"

- *Charaka Sutra 1/15*

moksha

Disclaimer

I am a certified, licenced, experienced nutrition consultant, an aesthetician, a cosmetologist, a wellness expert, a certified diabetic educator, nutrigenomics and gut health counsellor, obesity consultant, corporate nutritionist, public health advisor, blogger, writer, yoga practitioner, online support specialist, running my own brand *NutritionOnUrPlate* who has thoroughly reviewed medical claims, assertions, and recommendations for correctness and accuracy.

I have only used current and credible original sources, such as peer-reviewed medical journals, governmental organizations, educational institutions, and advocacy groups.

Please let us know if you see any inaccuracies or outdated information.

If you have a comment or a suggestion, please email us at NutritionOnUrPlate2020@gmail.com.

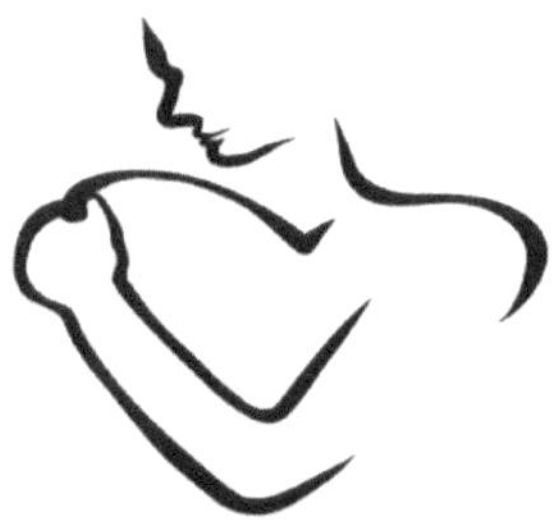

Testimonials

Had a lot of fun in exploring new dishes and enjoyed a lot while following your diet plans with agenda of *"No Diet"* diet ...Will surely catch up with u once everything is decided and I'm clear about how much time I'm having in following the plans. Till then thanks lot for your support and being ray of hope in the dark. ❣

- Anjali Haresh Alwani, Gandhidham, Kutch
Aspiring Doctor, MBBS Student

Enjoyed my sessions with my Preetha Kkiran a lot and really appreciate the knowledge she has and the help she gave me to look at things in a healthier way

- Deepali Singh
Banker U.A.E.

Preetha Kkiran also made me realize that meals don't need to be complicated and difficult; they can be fast and easy. Thanks so much for her help.

- Prafull Bhatt
VP, R &D, Multinational Company

I am here to share my amazing experience with you about Preetha Kkiran. What I love about her, I love her energy, her passion, and her simplicity. Her connection with traditional eating habits and traditional ways of cooking also helped me connect more. She doesn't only work on the food aspect but also your skin, hair, your workouts which will eventually help your stamina. She makes it simple yet interesting. So, if you are looking for a Nutritionist, you know where to go!

- Letitia George
Business Head, Healthcare

I am Rajnee Jain and I was gifted this program by my friend to work with Preetha Kkiran, especially during this lockdown time. I have had several complicated medical conditions- brain haemorrhage and a blood clot in the brain due to which my dietary needs are very specific as I am on blood thinners. One of the biggest challenges I was having was not able to exercise as I am not allowed to due to my condition. The good thing about working with Preetha was that I was able to regularize my eating habits and come to know what and when to eat. Although I did not lose a lot of weight as I did not commit to it long term. But in one month, I have managed to lose 3 kgs irrespective of my restrictions and I am able to follow up on all that I have learned during this time that is working wonders for me and I am getting the timely and right nutritional intake for my body. I am glad to have been part of this journey and all the best to Preetha I hope to get back to her soon and learn a lot more!

- *Rajnee Jain*
Events Management, U.A.E.

I thank my stars that I met her on an online platform randomly and especially when I was going through severe cystic acne and thyroid. I had no idea that these hormonal imbalances would bring various other issues in our body slowly and begin to damage. The concept of holistic lifestyle approach fell in place after I spoke to her and I had immediately enrolled in her program. It's more than 6 months now and I am super happy that I received what I asked for. She sets the plan based on clients need that features food plan, exercise, asanas, skin care and some Asian based practices that works wonders gradually. The food plans were great and doable, local and focused on tradition and what brought me more joy as I was allowed to eat everything in the right proportion. Preetha Kkiran is not only kind and warm and reaches out immediately to all my issues/ difficulties but she is one such person who will have your back at any given point. I have my share of bad days too and she is just a call away to vent out emotions, cry and be there and calm me down. Today if I have gained my flexibility when I am able to meditate for longer, maintain correct posture, sit in Starbucks and talk, or practice affirmations, my thyroid in control and better skin, it's all because of her. My deepest gratitude to Preetha Kkiran for bringing these holistic changes. I now know that balanced nutrition, discipline and exercise are key factors and with lifestyle changes, we can live healthier and a happy life. More love ❤ My first Nutritionist and forever.

- Zainab Malak
Puppet maker, Business Head, Mumbai

I feel that in today's world where nutritionists are very professional and in cut throat business, Preetha Kkiran has a kind of warmth in her, a very humane quality of reaching out and helping her clients in every way.

- Debjani Ghosh
Investment Advisor

Preetha has a very holistic approach when it comes to nutrition, eating homemade food and locally produced food. She believes in simplicity I feel and it reflects in her way of working with clients. She has a fantastic way of reaching out to you, talking to you, easing situations, and trying to adjust with the client's problems. She plans very simple, very homemade kind of food in her sessions which are really doable diets that produce fantastic results.

- Joyce D'Souza
Corporate Sector, U.A.E.

The plans are filled with a lot of nutrient rich food which gives you a lot of energy and she is a big advocate of yoga which is fantastic. I love the way she patiently explains about food and nutrition. She is very passionate of what she is doing and it reflects.

- Anjani Kiara
Owner, Trading Outlets, G.C.C.

Preetha Kkiran is a big motivation especially when I see her now filled with enthusiasm and energy to give her best. I love her work from home arrangements. Preetha is someone from whom I have personally learn a lot. She listens, she cares and she is awesome in all she is doing today.

-   Tasneem Kagzi
Baker, Owner Cloud Kitchen, Mumbai

I liked the process of systematically tracking the clients progress and your frequent reminder keeps one motivated all the time. With a total of 3 kgs weight loss and 3.9 inches lost. I have been taught that it's not just about the numbers but the whole process of maintaining this is by establishing a healthy relation with food. The best thing during my program was you always kept me informed about the diet and motivated me to gain knowledge of the food which I am eating instead of following it blindly which most of the dieticians generally do. I acquired so much knowledge on food, dieting and nutrition. And also liked the idea of inculcating a healthy diet into our lifestyle. I have no criticism...and I am really looking forward to asking your help again in future

-   Rashmi Kulkarni
Owner Sprouts Media, Web Designer

Always believe in the balanced Indian diet, which our family uses to follow and we use to have it in childhood. A BALANCED DIET is the primary factor in whatever you eat, you made me understand that. Always made me understand how to and what to order when we are going to a restaurant, never restrict me to eat outside but always taught me what to order. This is what is called a long-lasting diet plan which we can really learn after some time and carry our whole life. Thank you Preetha Kkiran not for the diet plan but for being my real mentor and friend. With whom defiantly lost weight but more than that I achieved a good lifestyle.

-   Biju & Shobha Pillai
Bankers/Professor, Management School

She is one of a kind and always has those encouraging words for you. Very understanding and never puts any pressure on you. On the contrary, I don't know how she does it but she motivates you to do better and to enjoy yourself in your sessions. I feel really privileged to have a person like her in my life. With her, you can achieve any goal, and I mean ANY!!!!! She is very professional and at the same time very friendly, she makes you feel like a part of the family. Thank you so much, Preetha for being such a wonderful person.

- *Sneha Lalwani*
Team Leader, International Trading

Preetha is incredibly responsive and I felt she is more like a food therapist than a dietician, which is exactly what I needed. I couldn't thank Preetha Kkiran enough. She helped me improve my mental health which made me feel so much better, simply because of her better nutrition advice. I would recommend everyone who's struggling to have a good diet please approach *NutritionOnUrPlate*

- *Priya Iyer*
Branch Head, International Banking

Witness your health transform as you walk along the simple facts and the power of the approach with the Intuitive Eating program that Preetha takes you through.

- *Raj Shekhar Reddy*
Founder NGO, Owner Hotel Chains Mumbai

A wonderful nutritionist. Very focused and has vast knowledge about her work and her diets are doable. She is also in tune with the medical world our health problems and how to overcome it by having a healthy diet. She is very caring and respects the condition of her clients we feel like we are her family, not clients. Her hard work, dedication, and efforts behind us make her a unique nutritionist. She is very responsive and plans and guides each session by making us understand what we are actually doing.

- Radha Ramakrishnan
Teacher

She is the best dietitian I have enrolled to; she really understands the wants and cravings perfectly and prepares a balanced meal plan for the same. Trust me guys, I enrolled for a weight gain programme and she has done wonders for me I highly recommend her for everyone looking for weight loss or gain or even just motivation.

- RJ Ved
Radio Jockey, Qatar

Preetha Kiran is wonderful and has helped me so much over the last year with eating and digestive issues. In addition to being a Nutritionist, she is like a mini-therapist–going beyond just "what did you eat" and really diving into the "whys" behind certain eating habits or symptoms I might be experiencing. She has done a wonderful job of meeting me where I am at and being non-judgemental and supportive throughout!

- Suneeta Kumble
Owner, Asmita Apparels (Designing Production House)

I'm so happy with the care I've received from *NutritionOnUrPlate*! I look forward to learning more and getting and staying healthier. Awesome team of providers!!! I have been trusting them with my nutritional goals for the past year and have learned so much. Their knowledge and patience are beyond measure. They are an incredible resource!

- Radhika & Prashant Joshi
Software Professional/Tour Organizer

We developed a great relationship, thanks to you for the lovely insights all along our association which turned in to a lifelong friendship, towards good health

- Dinesh Khiara
Owner – Khiara Traders U.A.E., GCC, India

What impressed me the most is the holistic way to lose weight with no side effects and constant motivation from Preetha and *her team*

\- *Sheetal Suresh*

Project Head Org Community Benefits, Africa

Transformation and learning with each day each step has made me an evolved individual, thank you Preetha Kkiran for this wonderful journey with you…

\- *Laredo Nell*

Owner Food Supply Chain, Philippines

References

Books

- Acharya Balkrishna (2016). A Practical Approach to the Science of Ayurveda: Bloomsbury

- Acharya Balkrishna (2018). A Sixteenth Century Ayurvedic Text on Food: Divya Prakashan

- Anuschka Rees (2019). Beyond Beautiful: Ten Speed Press

- B. Srilakshmi (2017). Nutrition Science: New Age International Publishers

- Emily Nagoski (2015). Come as You Are: Simon & Schuster

- Evelyn Tribole, Elyse Resch (2012). Intuitive Eating: St. Martin's Griffin

- Geneen Roth (2011). Women, Food and God: Scribner

- Janet Polivy, C. Peter Herman (1983). Breaking The Diet Habit: Basic Books

- Jenna Hollenstein (2019). Eat to Love: Lionheart Press

- K. R. Srikantha Murthy (1999). Astanga Samgraha of Vagbhata 6th Ed: Chaukhambha Orientalia

- Ken Albala, (2011). Food Cultures of the World Encyclopedia: Greenwood Press

- Laura Thomas (2019). Just Eat It: Bluebird

- Linda Bacon, Lindo Bacon (2010). Health At Every Size: BenBella Books

- Marion Nestle (2013). Food Politics: University Of California Press

- Meme Inge (2020). The Intuitive Eating Guide to Recovery: Rockridge Press

- Moly Groger (1986). Eating Awareness Training: Prentice Hall & IBD

- P. S. Sastri (2009). Text Book of Scientific Hindu Astrology Vol 1: Ranjan Publications

- P. V. Sharma (2005) Caraka Samhita: Chaukhambha Orientalia

- Rachael Hartley (2021). Gentle Nutrition: Victory Belt Publishing

- Rebecca Scritchfield (2017). Body Kindness: Workman Publishing

- Sanjeev Rastogi (2014). Ayurvedic Science of Food and Nutrition: Springer Nature

- William Benett, Joel Gurin (1983). Dieter's Dilemma: Basic Books

- Y. H. Hui (1983). Human Nutrition and Diet Therapy: Jones and Bartlett Publishers

Citations

- Aggett, P. J., Bresson, J., Haschke, F., Hernell, O., Koletzko, B., Lafeber, H. N., Michaelsen, K. F., Micheli, J., Ormisson, A., Rey, J., Salazar de Sousa, J., & Weaver, L. (1997). Recommended Dietary Allowances (RDAs), Recommended Dietary Intakes (RDIs), Recommended Nutrient Intakes (RNIs), and Population Reference Intakes (PRIs) are not "recommended intakes". Journal of pediatric gastroenterology and nutrition, 25(2), 236–241.

- Anderson, J. K. (2021). A brief Zoom-facilitated mindful and intuitive eating intervention to decrease disordered eating [Master's thesis, Minnesota State University, Mankato]. Cornerstone: A Collection of Scholarly and Creative Works for Minnesota State University, Mankato.

- Bashir, Hilal & Bhat, Shabir. (2016). Effects of Social Media on Mental Health: A Review. The International Journal of Indian Psychology. 4. 125 - 131. 10.25215/0403.134.

- Lew Louderback (1967). More people should be fat: Saturday Evening Post.

- Pradeepa, R., Anjana, R. M., Joshi, S. R., Bhansali, A., Deepa, M., Joshi, P. P., Dhandania, V. K., Madhu, S. V., Rao, P. V., Geetha, L., Subashini, R., Unnikrishnan, R., Shukla, D. K., Kaur, T., Mohan, V., Das, A. K., & ICMR-INDIAB Collaborative Study Group (2015). Prevalence of generalized & abdominal obesity in urban & rural India--the ICMR-INDIAB Study (Phase-I) [ICMR- NDIAB-3]. The Indian journal of medical research, 142(2), 139–150.

- Rastogi, Sanjeev. (2013). Ayurvedic Principles of Food and Nutrition: Translating Theory into Evidence-Based Practice. Ayurvedic Science of Food and Nutrition. 3-14. 10.1007/978-1-4614-9628-1_1.

- Vaidyanathan, S., Kuppili, P. P., & Menon, V. (2019). Eating Disorders: An Overview of Indian Research. Indian journal of psychological medicine, 41(4), 311–317.

www.ingramcontent.com/pod-product-compliance
Lightning Source LLC
Chambersburg PA
CBHW051305250726
48656CB00004B/1479